"This is an important and interesting book since it addresses the problems associated with women's mental health in Africa apart from those of men, which has not been done before in one volume. The contributors cover a wide range of issues, from spirit possession to AIDS, in a sympathetic and scholarly manner. It should be read by all those involved in medical and paramedical fields and by concerned lay people."

Georgina Buijs, PhD, Lecturer, Department of Anthropology, Rhodes University, Grahamstown, South Africa

Women's Mental Health in Africa

Women's Mental Health in Africa

Edited by
Esther D. Rothblum and Ellen Cole

Women's Mental Health in Africa was simultaneously issued by The Haworth Press, Inc., under the same title, as a special issue of *Women & Therapy*, Volume 10, Number 3 1990, Esther D. Rothblum and Ellen Cole, Editors.

Harrington Park Press
New York • London

ISBN 0-918393-86-8

Published by

Harrington Park Press, 10 Alice Street, Binghamton, NY 13904-1580
EUROSPAN/Harrington, 3 Henrietta Street, London WC2E 8LU England

Harrington Park Press is a subsidiary of The Haworth Press, Inc., 10 Alice Street, Binghamton, NY 13904-1580.

Women's Mental Health in Africa was originally published as *Women & Therapy*, Volume 10, Number 3 1990.

Cover design by Marshall Andrews.

Library of Congress Cataloging-in-Publication Data

Women's mental health in Africa / edited by Esther D. Rothblum and Ellen Cole.
        p. cm.
        "Simultaneously issued by the Haworth Press, Inc., under the same title, as a special issue of Women & therapy, volume 10, number 3, 1990."
        Includes bibliographical references.
        ISBN 0-918393-86-8 (alk. paper)
        1. Women — Mental health — Africa. 2. Women — Africa — Psychology. I. Rothblum, Esther D. II. Cole, Ellen.
        [DNLM: 1. Mental Health. 2. Sociology, Medical — Africa. 3. Women — psychology. WA 305 W8729]
RC451.4.W6W666 1990
362.2'082 — dc20
DNLM/DLC
for Library of Congress   90-5363
                                                                                                                            CIP

CONTENTS

ABOUT THE EDITORS

Esther D. Rothblum, PhD, is Associate Professor in the department of psychology at the University of Vermont. She is currently a Kellogg Fellow and has travelled to Africa to study women's mental health. Her research and writing have focused on mental health disorders in which women predominate, including depression, the social stigma of women's weight, procrastination and fear of failure, and women in the Antarctic. She has co-edited six books, including *Another Silenced Trauma: Twelve Feminist Therapists and Activists Respond to One Woman's Recovery From War*, which received a 1987 Distinguished Publication Award from the Association for Women in Psychology. Dr. Rothblum is a co-editor of the journal *Women & Therapy* and co-editor of the Haworth Series on Women.

Ellen Cole, PhD, has devoted 25 years to the practice of psychology. She is currently an adjunct faculty member in the Human Development Program, Prescott College, Prescott, Arizona. An AASECT certified sex therapist and sex educator, she was formerly a professor of psychology at Goddard College in Vermont and chair of the Committee on Women and Minorities of the Vermont Psychological Association. In addition, she co-edited, with Esther Rothblum, the book *Another Silenced Trauma*, which received a 1987 Distinguished Publication Award from the Association for Women in Psychology. Dr. Cole is a co-editor of the journal *Women & Therapy* and co-editor of the Haworth Series on Women.

Gender and Mental Health in Africa

Mere Nakateregga Kisekka

GENDER DIFFERENCES

Two assumptions underlie the study of gender differences: the biological one which looks for genetic gender-linked predisposing factors, and the sociological one which regards gender-roles as psychodynamically important in the etiology of mental illnesses. Following the latter assumption, we note that men and women are exposed to different strains and stresses and employ divergent coping mechanisms and compensatory resources and hence suffer from varying psychiatric morbidity.

Available studies of admissions to psychiatric institutions unequivocally report higher rates for men than women. Thus, in a prospective study of 372 consecutive admissions in seven and a half weeks, in 1968 at Butabika Hospital in Uganda, Orley (1972) counted 247 males in comparison to 125 females. In reference to researches elsewhere, Orley reports that Carothers, in a five year period (1939-43) in a series of 558 consecutive admissions of Kenya Africans in Mathari Mental Hospital, established a ratio of two men to one woman. Smartt is also quoted as having, in 1954, examined 252 mental patients admitted to Mirembe Hospital in Tanzania and to have arrived at the ratio of 2.8 men to 1 woman. In

The author is a Ugandan lecturer engaged in teaching and research in Nigeria since 1974, in the areas of medical sociology, social psychology and women's studies. She is a past Vice President of the Association of African Women for Research and Development (1983-1988) and the current national coordinator of the Women's Health Network in Nigeria.

This is the author's revised paper of "Psychocultural stress and African women" *African Journal of Mental Health and Society*, 1981, *1*(1); 44-59.

Requests for reprints may be sent to Dr. Mere Kisekka, Dept. Sociology, Ahmadu Bello University, Zaria, Nigeria.

1

South Africa, Orley cites a researcher who in a period of ten years, at Queenstown Mental Hospital, encountered 670 male and 419 female admissions. Then in Ghana at the Accra Psychiatric Hospital, Lamptey (1977) put the male to female ratio at 2 to 1. In Sierra Leone, at the Kissy Mental Hospital in Freetown, Dawson (1964) put the sex ratio at 2.58 males to each female. Altogether these reports are strikingly consistent in their estimation of a preponderance of men over women in hospitalization rates.

One is led then to speculate over the causes of these gender differentials in rates of hospitalization. For one thing, men are dominant in the formal employment sectors where they enjoy free medicare and other employment benefits and are therefore likely to be referred to hospitals for treatment. Secondly, not only are men more physically aggressive than women, but they predominate among city marginals and consequently they are easily exposed to mandated caretakers, particularly the police. This last point is corroborated by Orley (1970) who showed that in a breakdown of admissions for the months of October 1967 and April 1969 at Butabika Hospital in Uganda, the difference in admission figures between males and females was most obvious in cases coming from police stations.

The last point to account for gender differences in rates of admissions has to do with the fact that women are exposed and oriented to the use of alternative facilities such as spiritual churches and indigenous traditional healers. So, perhaps if epidemiological surveys were taken, a different picture of gender variations might emerge. Thus Benite (1977) quotes that in a survey of 65 villages among the Serer Senegal, with a population of 35,000, Beiser found 10 males and 20 females with psychiatric disorders. However, Leighton, Lambo, and Hughes (1963) in a survey of Yoruba, asserted that women in general had fewer psychiatric symptoms and better mental health than men.

With regard to gender variations in symptomatology, it is unfortunate that we have even fewer studies dealing with the issue. Nevertheless, there seems to be an indication that there is gender patterning in relation to neurotic, psychosomatic, affective and conduct disorders. Thus among others, studies of Ebie (1972) and Odejide (1981) in Nigeria, and that of Otsyula and Rees (1972) in

Kenya, all show higher incidence of depression and psychosomatic disorders among females than males. The Leighton, Lambo, and Hughes (1963) study is however an exception in reporting a greater prevalence of psychoneurotic symptoms among Yoruba men than their female counterparts. But as for conduct disorders, particularly alcoholism and drug addiction, they are as reported so far, male dominated diseases.

WOMEN'S MENTAL ILLNESSES

This section focuses on psychiatrically screened symptoms and their variation with women's social characteristics. The irony though is that there are merely a handful of such studies and as such they deserve detailed discussion.

In Nigeria, a study conducted by Murphy (1965) was summarized as: "A systematic epidemiological study of 156 non-literate Yoruba women and 120 English-speaking Yoruba women indicates that the modern Yoruba women have a higher prevalence of psychoneurotic and psychosomatic disorders but that increase is not statistically significant." In the same country, Ebie (1976) studied records of 1391 female psychiatric patients over a seven year period (1963-71). The characteristics of these patients were as follows: 66 per cent were married while 25 per cent were single and the rest were previously married; the age groups most represented were 21-30 years (39 per cent) and 31-40 years (26 per cent). With respect to symptoms, 60 percent suffered from psychoses, mostly of the schizophrenic type.

The relationship between women's mental health and pregnancy (as distinct from the puerperium) has been explored in Uganda (Assael & Namboze, 1972). The authors noted that women attending antenatal clinics tended to want to discuss their domestic and social problems even when no questions were asked. This behavior did not characterize non-antenatal patients. Then in a random sample of 100 antenatal patients, 24 were found with conspicuous psychiatric disturbance, mainly depression of a psychogenic or reactive type. This group of psychiatric patients was found to have differed significantly from the rest in the random sample in that they either lived alone, were co-wives or had in the past suffered traumatic deliveries like caesarean section, stillbirth or difficult labor. The authors explained that although the problems the patients complained about were understandable and believable, they were nevertheless exaggerated and charged with great emotional tension. These problems, which mostly centered on co-wives and antagonism with the husband, were expressed in paranoid reaction (10 patients) and anxiety (6 patients). Paranoia culminated in increased belief in magic and witches and led to a search for traditional doctors and diviners. As for anxiety, it was revealed in fears, loss of peace, and dizziness — all of which were related to pregnancy, childbirth, poverty, housing, and family problems.

The authors, two of them medical doctors including a Ugandan woman (J. Namboze) and the other a psychiatrist, note that the incidence of mental disturbance in this group (24 per cent) was excessively high and above the prevalence rate in the East African population generally. They further speculate that if, as in developed countries, 14 per cent of all serious mental disorders in women are related to reproduction and childbirth, in Africa this situation must be exacerbated in view of the high fertility rates and the considerably worse economic and medical plight.

Yet, another equally revealing study conducted in Ghana (Danquah, 1978), deals specifically with psychoneuroses as related to women's social problems. The study was motivated by the observation that women formed a majority of patients suffering from depression both as out-patients and in-patients. This was later confirmed in a two-year investigation of a community of nearly one million people near Accra. It was found that out of 11,298 people identified in psychiatric and traditional healing units as suffering from psychoneuroses, 53 per cent were females, mostly from lower socio-economic classes. Then on the basis of questionnaire and interview schedules from 5,132 psychoneurotic patients, the highest rates were found among those who had attained some degree of college and university education, followed by those with no formal schooling.

With respect to social problems, the greatest number (69 per cent) emanated from the home environment, mainly sexual problems (i.e., anorgasmia and sexual dissatisfaction), husband's inability to provide sufficient housekeeping money, and his objectionable behavior in wife-beating and alcoholism. However, infidelity, in-laws, co-wives, and social neglect did not figure high in the list of perceived marital problems. The second category of problems was in connection with jobs and was expressed in terms of discrimination and sexual overtures from male colleagues.

Now, when we turn to postpartum or puerperal mental illness we find that it is one disorder that has received quite some attention from clinicians in various parts of the continent. To begin with, puerperal mental illness is defined as a disorder that occurs during the first year after a woman has delivered, but some researchers limit it to only three or six months. The illness is not different from other mental disorders except for the speculation that chemical changes or psychological stress of childbirth might be of etiological significance in its occurrence.

In a discussion of research on puerperal psychosis by clinicians in Africa, Swift and Asuni (1975) note that all the studies have been retrospective and that all the patients involved had developed their problems two weeks after delivery. In about half of the women studied, there was a febrile illness during the puerperium, while in the rest postpartum hemorrhage or toxaemia of pregnancy had occurred. Additionally, they observe that a small number of the women are reported to have revealed, on examination, gross malnutrition, vitamin deficiency (pellegra), hypertension, or epilepsy. Elsewhere, Swift (1972) comments that these findings are in dramatic contrast with those of Euro-America where the leading diagnosis among women's puerperal psychiatric illness is affective disorders.

Another project which reports on puerperal psychoses is a field study conducted by an anthropologist for thirteen months among the Loma of Liberia. Prince (1976), who reviews this work, quotes the anthropologist as having asserted that 73 per cent of psychoses among women occurred in the postpartum period as opposed to the 8-12 per cent found in some western societies.

PSYCHOSOCIAL STRESS AND WOMEN'S STRAIN

Strictly speaking, the words strain and stress connote different meanings. But in common usage, they, together with others like tension and pressure, are simultaneously applied to environmental forces impinging on individuals, as well as their reactions to those forces (Langner & Michael, 1963). But in the true psychological sense, stress can be regarded as any noxious stimulus, while strain is the individual's psychic cost or response to stress.

There are many events and conditions which can be described as stressful. They may be economic, like unemployment or poverty; physical ones, like sickness or fatigue; or simply psychological, like bereavement or neglect. Such stressful events may be seen as the immediate and intermediate causes, or to put it another way, predisposing and precipitating factors of mental illness. Strain, or mental and bodily reaction to stress, can result in disordered behavior characterized by anxiety or psychophysiological changes.

However, regarding the relationship between stress and development of psychiatric disorders, Schwab and Schwab (1978) rightly caution that it is clinically evident but scientifically elusive. For while in some cases stressful events precede the onset of mental illness and thus appear to have caused significance, in other instances people break down mentally when there is little indication that their lives have been stressful.

Notwithstanding those inconsistencies, feminist researchers are very concerned with at least two sets of stressful events for African women. One set of factors emanates from the traditional cultural values, taboos and prescriptions which are inimical to women's self-concept as well as physical health. The second set of factors revolves around structural changes resulting from the modernization processes which have marginalized women and reaped them disbenefits.

The culturally stressful psycho-social factors that have aroused most attention concern sex and reproduction (AAWORD, 1979). Certain sexual practices like clitoridectomy and infibulation have been associated with problems ranging from vaginal fistulae, genital infections leading to infertility and severe problems at childbirth, to lack of sexual response. Regarding reproduction, problems are created for women when they have no children at all, have too many or fail to have the desired number and sex.

First, one must note the excessive stigma attached to barrenness, despite the cultural alternative of child fostering. Both traditional and modern folklore, literature and popular music are replete with depictions of barren women as lonely, malicious, cruel to children and always coveting and bewitching other peoples' children. The modern alternative of attaining social and emotional fulfillment through carccr aspirations is, understandably, as yet utopian to the majority of women. It is therefore not surprising that barren women tend to feature prominently in the supernaturalistic roles of diviners and prophetesses. Similarly, the high valuation placed on children also explains the lack of social stigma attached to unmarried parenthood. For, according to one male Yoruba psychiatrist, "in the ultimate being a parent is the higher status symbol than being childless in a marriage" (Ayonrinde, 1976).

High, and in many cases, unspaced fertility is also a common expectation and experience. In fact, there is sometimes little differentiation made between a woman who has one or two children and one who has none at all. For many women, the average desired family size is anywhere between eight and twelve children. The conflict involving on the one hand in the emotional and physical strain, and on the other the internalized values of having such a large family are not infrequently resolved by the development of psychosomatic disorders (Ayorinde, 1976). The knowledge that men can always get a second wife or beget children from "outside" women, compels even those women who want small families, for economic or medical reasons, to produce more children simply to avert their husbands' "beyond the marriage" approach. In the case of an already neo- or polygamous marriage, there is an element of competition in the reproductive values and behavior of women. In any case, regardless of the type of marriage, a large family size is regarded as a measure of marital success, happiness and future economic security.

Equally stressful are certain beliefs associated with difficult deliveries and miscarriages. It is usually believed that these events are caused by a woman's illicit sexual relations, and therefore necessitate a confession of guilt on her part. Also, among many groups, birth of twins generates severe maternal anxiety. Such stressful beliefs may contribute to postpartum psychiatric illness and other psychophysiological and anxiety symptoms associated with pregnancy and childbirth.

Ironically, at the opposite extreme is the increasing number of women who suffer the burden of unwanted pregnancies: this is mainly because these pregnancies are career contingencies as they result in expulsion from schools or jobs, or when the women involved lack independent and feasible means to maintain themselves. The situation of such women is exacerbated by the restrictive and unsecular approach to abortion and modern contraception that occurs in many of the African countries today. The psychological trauma that accompanies these unwanted pregnancies is revealed in the increasing rates of young women's suicides, abandonment of babies and cases of infanticide. Suicide rates thus seem to be higher among women than men, and are associated generally with an increase in education and absence of strong traditional support in the cities.

The association between mental health and those issues of sexuality and reproduction is validated, both impressionistically and empirically, in the utilization of spiritual churches and traditional healers. Women, who are the main users of these facilities, go there to seek magico-religious cures for genito-urinary problems, infertility, and other problems connected with childbirth and sexual functioning (Devish, 1977; Ngubane, 1976; Uyanga, 1979). Similarly, Bohannan's classical book *African Homicide and Suicide* (1960) confirms the centrality of sexual and reproductive issues in the etiology of women's suicides.

Another area of life, saturated with stressful conditions for women, is work and employment. Much of the stress is the result of "disbenefits" of the modernization processes such as commercialization of land, monetization of agriculture and reform. Justice cannot be done here to explicate these issues, which have become the major focus of study in the women and development literature (Tadesse, 1980); it is sufficient to merely highlight their deleterious effects on women's mental health.

In the first instance, in the rural areas, women's socio-economic positions have deteriorated or stagnated in comparison to the premodernization days. Thus, perennial cash crops have become institutionalized as male crops, while women as the chief cultivators of food crops have become unpaid family workers on men's farms (Hanger & Morris, 1973; Pala, 1979). Systematically too, the new technologies in farming, farm inputs and credit extension have ignored women, increased their labor demand and created wide income differentials between the sexes (Akerele, 1979; Boserup, 1970). Lastly, the male-dominated migration from rural to urban areas (Youssef, Buvinic & Kudat, 1979) has contributed to an increasing matrifocality, making women the "primary" reproducers of labor.

In the urban areas, women predominate in the low-level industrial jobs, in the informal sector, prostitution and other exploitative relationships. Variously in these positions, women suffer a number of constraints: lack of unemployment benefits and credit facilities (Lewis, 1978); legal inferiority; prejudice and discrimination against entrepreneurial and proprietary control (Gutto, 1976); "invisible underemployment"; unconducive environmental conditions and exploitation by middlemen; lack of prospects for on-the-job training, and hence of career mobility; as well as non-availability of institutional facilities for maternal employment (Tadesse, 1976; United National Economic Commission for Africa/African Training Research Center for Women, 1973). Altogether, it has been shown in Palmer's (1979) review of the International Labor Organization report in Kenya, that female migrants and household heads constitute some of the most economically depressed segments of the urban population; these findings can probably be replicated in most of the African countries.

Last but not least are the increasing incidences of sexual harassment in schools and workplaces by both colleagues and male bosses. The structural adjustment policies with their stringent fiscal policies have resulted in massive unemployment and retrenchment of workers, a situation which has put so much pressure on women as victims of exploitative sexual liaisons in their bid not to jeopardize their precarious economic situations.

Likewise, the extensive and prolonged internal civil strife in many of the African countries has made military rule the order of the day, often accompanied by brutal sexual aggression.

In other places women's genitals are frequently used in ritualistic ceremonies and as such women become targets of kidnap, sexual molestation, and sacrifice.

RESEARCH QUESTIONS

A number of issues discussed in this paper need more systematic investigation than that which has been undertaken to date. First of all, we need information at the descriptive level regarding the variation of psychiatric problems with women's socio-demographic characteristics. For example, how is neurosis spread among women of different ages, socio-economic and marital levels, etc.?

Secondly, at a more analytical level we can look at the relationship between gender-role stressful events and mental illness. Here, one needs to investigate both among psychiatric patients and matched controls of non-psychiatric patients. Among the most commonly hypothesized stressful situations in the African environment are: barrenness, failure to have the desired number and sex of children, unwanted pregnancies, divorces, matrifocality, and early and forced marriages.

The third area of research concerns the relationship between socio-economic environmental factors and women's mental health. That is, for example, the effect on mental health of living in urban versus rural areas, or living in a racist environment, or in a community of high male out-migration.

Last but not least is the issue of gender differences. One of the intriguing lines of investigation is to find out how much of the Euro-American findings can be replicated, or whether gender reversals do occur. These findings can go a long way in illuminating the debate over the relative influences of nature versus nurture in mental health, in terms of subjective self-evaluation. Are African married men better off mentally than their married women counterparts? With regard to children, how do such events as impotence or inability to have the desired number and gender of children affect African men in comparison to women?

Altogether, the field of mental health of women in Africa is virgin. It is replete with some of the most provocative feminist issues of the day. Methodologically, we have to do epidemiological studies in communities and treatment facilities. There is need for prospective as well as retrospective work. Autobiographical descriptions of subjective stress and strain recounted by ex-patients and non-patients can throw light on "the definition of situation" and hence the various coping and compensatory mechanisms which create adjustment or maladjustment. Research can be carried out by social scientists alone, but perhaps more fruitfully in collaboration with psychiatric personnel like doctors and social workers. For comparable and meaningful research, the designs, measurement instruments and indices have to be standardized.

Ultimately, the hope of such research undertakings is that inimical situations to the mental health of women can be clearly and early identified so as to demand prompt and just preventive and therapeutic measures.

REFERENCES CITED

Akerele, O. (1979). Women and the fishing industries in Liberia, *Economic Commission for Africa/African Training*. Research Center for Women, Addis Ababa, Ethiopia.

Assael, M.I., & Namboze, J. (1972). Psychiatric disturbances during pregnancy in a rural group of African women. *Social Science and Medicine*, *6*, 387-395.

Association of African Women for Research and Development (1979). Genital mutilation: A statement by AAWORD. Presented to the second Regional Conference on the Integration of Women in Development, Lusaka, Zambia.

Ayorinde, A. (April, 1976). Marriage, family planning and mental health status of Nigerian women. Paper presented at the National Conference on Nigerian Women and Development. University of Ibadan, Nigeria.

Benite, A. (1977). Patterns of psychiatric care in African countries. *Nigerian Medical Journal*, June 34-39.

Bohannan, P. (1960). *African Homicide and Suicide*. Princeton, NJ: Princeton University Press.

Boserup, E. (1970). *Women's Role in Economic Development*. London, England: Allen and Unwin.

Danquah, S.A., (September, 1978). Some aspects of mental health of Ghanain women: Female psychoneuroses and social problems. Paper presented at Women Development Seminar, Trinity College, Legon, Ghana.

Dawson, J. (1964). Urbanization and mental health in a West African community. In A. Kiev (Ed.), *Magic, Faith and Healing*. New York: The Free Press.

Devisch, R. (1977). Processes for the articulation of meaning and ritual healing among the Northern Yaka (Zaire). *Anthropos*, 72 683-708.

Ebie, J.C. (1972). Some observations on depressive illness in Nigerians attending a psychiatric out-patients clinic. *African Journal of Medical Science*, *3*, 14-155.

Ebie, J.C. (1976). A review of patients admitted to the female psychiatric ward of a university college hospital in Nigeria. *Nigerian Medical Journal*, 79-83.

Gutto, S.B.O. (1976). The status of women in Kenya: A study of paternalism, inequality and underprivilege. Discussion Paper No. 235, Institute for Development Studies University of Nairobi, Nairobi, Kenya.

Hanger, I., & Morris, J. (1973). Women and the household economy. In R. Chamber and J. Morris (Eds.). *Mwea: An irrigated rice settlement in Kenya*. Munich, West Germany: Weltforum Verlag.

Langner, T.S., & Michael, S.T. (1963). *Life Stress and Mental Health*. London: The Free Press of Glencoe.

Lamptey, J.J. (1977). Patterns of psychiatric consultations at the Accra Psychiatric Hospital. *African Journal of Psychiatry*, *3*, 123-127.

Leighton, A.H., Lambo, T.A., & Hughes, C.C. (1963). *Psychiatric disorders among the Yoruba*. Ithaca, NY: Cornell University Press.

Lewis, B.C. (1978). The limitation of group action among entrepreneurs: The market women of Abidjan, Ivory Coast. In N. J. Hafkin (Ed.), *Women in Africa*. Palo Alto, CA: University Press.

Murphy, J.M. (1965). Cultural change and mental health among Yoruba women of Nigeria. Paper presented at African Studies Association Annual Meeting.

Ngubane, H. (1976). Some aspects of treatment among the Zulu. In J.B. London, (Ed.), *Social Anthropology and Medicine*. London: Academic Press.

Odejide, O.A. (1981). Chronic psychiatric patients in Nigeria: Factors predicting chronicity and militating against successful rehabilitation. Paper presented at First Regional Conference: Social Science and Mental Health Planning in Africa, Ibadan, Nigeria.

Orley, J. (1970). *Culture and mental illness: A study from Uganda*. Nairobi, Kenya: East African Publishing House.

Orley, J. (1972). A prospective study of 372 consecutive admissions to Butabika Hospital, Kampala. *East African Medical Journal*, ·'9, 16-26.

Otsyula, W., & Rees, P.H. (1972). The occurrence and recognition of minor psychiatric illness among outpatients at Kenyatta National Hospital, Nairobi. *East African Medical Journal*, *49*, 825-829.

Pala, A.O. (1979). *African women in rural development: Research trends and priorities*. Overseas Liaison Committee Paper 12, Washington, D.C.

Palmer, I. (1979). New official ideas on women and development. *Institute for Development Studies* (IDS) *10*, 42-52.

Prince, R. (1976). Culture and psychoses among the Loma Tribe of Liberia, West Africa. *African Journal of Psychiatry, 3*, 381-383.

Schwab, J.J., & Schwab, M.E. (1978). *Sociocultural roots of mental illness*. New York: Plenum Medical Book Co.

Swift, C.R. (1972). Psychosis during the reurperium among Tanzanians. *East African Medical Journal*, *49*, 652-657.

Swift, C.R., & Asuni, T. (1975). *Mental health and disease in Africa*. London: Churchill Livingston.

Tadesse, Z. (1976). The conditions of women in Ethiopia. Report to Swedish International Development Agency.

Tadesse, Z. (May 1980). Research trends on women in Subsaharan Africa. Paper presented to UNESCO Meeting of Experts on Research and Teaching Related to Women: Evaluation and Prospects, Paris, France.

UNECA/ATRCW (1979). Women textile workers in Ethiopia. Unpublished manuscript. Addis Ababa, Ethiopia.

Uyanga, J. (1979). The characteristics of patients of spiritual healing homes and traditional doctors in South-Eastern Nigeria. *Social Science and Medicine*, *13A*, 323-329.

Youssef, N., Buvinic, M., & Kudat, A. (1979). Women in migration: A Third World Focus by International Center for Research on Women. Office of Women in Development, Washington, DC.

Mental Health Aspects of Zar for Women in Sudan

Edith H. Grotberg

SUMMARY. Zar, an ancient cult of northern Africa, has developed in the Sudan and addresses many of the mental health problems of Sudanese women. The continuing and increasing participation in Zar ceremonies by Sudanese women probably results from the effectiveness of Zar as it is adapted to the unique needs of Sudanese women. The effectiveness of Zar is consistent with the effectiveness of mental health programs around the world, and, indeed, incorporates the universal concepts and assumptions of most successful mental health treatment programs. The universal concepts and assumptions are: (1) the client recognizes something is wrong and seeks help; (2) a theory is available to explain the problem; and (3) a therapy is used which includes a trusted leader, assumptions of client guiltlessness, a ritual of meetings and actions, and expected results.

The Zar ceremony draws upon each of these concepts and assumptions, with the sheikha (priestess) being the leader, the blameless victim possessed by an evil spirit, a ritual of dancing, incense, etc., and satisfactory results in mental health status. Social changes and upheavals, particularly rural to urban movement, seem to account for the continuing and increasing participation of Sudanese women in Zar ceremonies.

Dr. Edith H. Grotberg is currently Senior Associate for the Institute for Mental Health Initiatives, Washington, DC. She continues to maintain her professional affiliation with Ahfad University for Women, Omdurman, Sudan. Dr. Grotberg, a psychologist, was formerly Director of the Research Division of the Administration for Children, Youth and Families, the Department of Health and Human Services, Washington, DC.

Reprinted with permission from *The Ahfad Journal: Women and Change*, 1985, 2(2), 28-35.

Requests for reprints may be sent to Dr. Edith Grotberg, #1216, 4141 N. Henderson Rd., Arlington, VA 22203.

15

INTRODUCTION

The mental health aspects of Zar for women in Sudan are best understood by examining the cult against some universal concepts and assumptions found in most treatments of mental health problems. These universal concepts and assumptions vary from place to place, culture to culture, and with different kinds of knowledge, but the variations seem more adaptations than disparates.

A brief identification of universal concepts and assumptions in treatment of mental health problems provides a backdrop to examining their adaptation to Sudan culture in general and to the subculture of Sudanese women in particular.

The universal concepts and assumptions in treatment of mental health problems are:

1. The client recognizes something is wrong and seeks help;
2. A theory is available to explain the problem; and
3. A therapy is used which includes:

   a. a leader who is trusted, provides confidential interpersonal exchange, and is seen as having special powers and authority;
   b. assumptions that the client is not guilty, but more a blameless victim, and the client can be helped;
   c. a ritual which includes:

      (1) schedule times and prepared places for meetings;
      (2) individual talks and/or group discussions; and
      (3) specific actions to be taken by the client and those around the client;

   d. results which alleviate the problem or help the client live with it, controlling the more destructive aspects.

Zar as practiced among women in Sudan is described within the framework of these universal concepts and assumptions, recognizing the adaptations made to Sudanese cultures.

THE CULT OF ZAR

Zar is found throughout northern and western Sudan, in Ethiopia, in tribes of West Africa and Somalia and into Egypt and Arabia, and also into Libya, Tunisia and throughout the Sahara. The cult originated in Ethiopia and was associated with a sky god, later degenerating into an evil spirit. In the Sudan, Zar has become a semi-religious cult involving women primarily. The Zar cult consists of spirit possession, initially regarded as an illness, and ranges from depression and infertility to actual organic and psychological disorders. According to Cloudsley (1983, p. 75), "these disturbances are attributed to hostile spirits, demons or jinn. Zar is the name given to the ceremony required to pacify spirits known as *zar, dustur,* or *rihahmar.*"

Zar ceremonies are still popular in the Sudan and recent research indicates an increase in Zar adherents over the last decade. This increase is attributed in part to major social upheavals resulting from rural to urban migrations (Ayton, 1984). The increase occurs in spite of opposition to it by the more educated or more devout Muslims. In fact, in recent research, Nemat-Mubarak (1985) found that more literate (62%) than illiterate (38%) women attended Zar ceremonies and more middle and upper class (59%) women than lower class (41%) women participate. These were women from the metropolitan area of Khartoum. The reasons for continuing Zar ceremonies certainly include the effectiveness of the ceremonies for many women and, as becomes clear upon describing the various aspects of Zar, its remarkable acceptability to the unique needs of Sudanese women.

THE PRACTICE OF ZAR

The practice of Zar in Sudan is described according to the universal concepts and assumptions in treatment of mental health problems as well as to adaptations to specific Sudanese cultural features.

1. *Recognition of problem.* Sudanese women talk among themselves a great deal, particularly with the female members of the family. These conversations, primarily social in nature, include discussion of feelings, concerns, and persistent or emerging problems.

From these conversations, a woman who seems particularly troubled and is depressed or in pain, may decide she, indeed, has a problem and needs help. She may agree to accompany others to a Zar ceremony, or she may decide to have a Zar especially for herself. If she is married, her husband is expected to cover the expenses. However, recent research (Nemat-Mubarak, 1985), using a population of 100 women from the metropolitan area of Khartoum who participated in Zar ceremonies, indicates that only 9% of the women are married, while 20% are divorced, 35% are widowed, and 39% are unmarried. It is not clear who provides the money to these women.

2. *Available theory for cause of problem*. Zar, as a very old cult, has formulated a basic theory to explain women's problems. The problems result, according to the theory, from possession by a spirit and a person so possessed is slave to the spirit and must do its bidding. This basic theory becomes flexible in terms of which spirits possess which women and introduces the notion of status. To illustrate, there are six human spirits of the Zar cult, represented in Zar by four different flags as follows:

Beshir El Habashi, an Ethiopian Christian spirit who is of primary importance; represented by a red flag; Bernawi, an Ethiopian Muslim; represented by a black flag; Bendawi, an African spirit, shares red flag with Beshir; Sheikh Abdel Gadir el Gailani, an Arab Muslim; represented by a white flag; Bilal, a spirit from the Bernou tribe of Nigeria; represented by a green flag; and Tournberani, a spirit of a white Christian; shares the black flag.

It should be noted that the spirits are all of men only. There is much confusion about which spirit was from where and there is frequent introduction of new spirits, again reflecting flexibility and adaptability to changing needs and conditions.

According to Samia El Hadi el Nagar (1978), these spirits were under the influence of the Prophet Suleiman. They appeared before him and when he ordered them to descend, they refused. However, they said they could be influenced by the smell of incense and the rhythms of drums. They also said they were capable of troublesome possession and would only leave humans alone if they were honored with singing, dancing, and trappings of luxury.

The list of spirits is in terms of priority of importance and Beshir

seems to be the main possessor and is the most importa.
Women possessed are not possessed by these spirits, but only
spirits of animals or other low ranking beings. The powerful s₊
which are present at all Zar occasions only possess the priest
herself as she attempts to remove the lesser spirits from a possesser
client.

3. *Therapy*. The features of therapy, consistent with mental
health practice, are described as follows:

a. A leader. The leader in the Zar cult is a priestess, called sheikha, who is drawn into the cult by an overwhelming sense of voca-
tion. Further, she must have overcome a serious illness herself to
assure others that the spirits associated with her have curative abili-
ties. She has an understanding with the spirits and can diagnose
cases of spirit possession. She is selected by a client mainly for her
reputation. The sheikha may have assistants, some of whom were
beneficiaries of previous Zars, but the sheikha is the dominant force
and is the only one who can deal with the spirits.

b. Guiltlessness. The spirits possessing women are considered to
be amoral. They are perceived to strike entirely capriciously and
without reference to the moral character or conduct of the victims.
However, they are not totally indiscriminate as they usually choose
the down-trodden and the weak, i.e., women. By succumbing to
such spirits, underprivileged and oppressed individuals find relief
and attract attention to themselves without carrying a burden of
guilt. Women so possessed cannot help themselves, nor are they
blamed for the cost of the treatment. Responsibility lies entirely
with the spirits. The victim is helpless and must do the bidding of
the spirit.

c. The ritual. The Zar ritual is described in three phases:

(1) Scheduled time and prepared place. The sheikha and client
may agree on the time and place for the Zar ceremony; however,
there are a variety of fixed dates for holding Zar ceremonies. One is
the month of Rajab which includes the Muslim festival of the Night
of Decree. Ceremonies are also held on other religious occasions,
especially the Prophet's birthday. Large scale Zar meetings are held
just before Ramadan, as during Ramadan there are no meetings
because the spirits are believed to be rendered inactive by the will of
God.

In addition to Zar meetings scheduled by the sheikha and a client and those scheduled on religious dates, are a series of less formal Zar meetings held on Wednesday and Saturday of each week. These are seen as "blessing" ceremonies and revolve around the use of bakhoor (incense) and the freedom to discuss intimate problems with the sheikha. These meetings are attended by many women who have come to be cured of minor spiritual ailments or who have brought relatives to be cured. Each of the clients pays a small amount of money for the consultation.

There is no precise starting time for a Zar ceremony; rather it starts when a sufficient number of people arrive or when the sheikha decides to start. There is no clear termination time either; however, Nemat-Mubarak (1985) found that the ceremony can last from one to seven days, with three the usual length.

Preparations for Zar ceremonies include clearing and sweeping an area and providing carpets for dancing and a decorated canopy to protect the dancers from the sun. Around the dancing area are hung four flags placed in metal cans containing gravel. These stand against the wall and a bowl of burning incense is placed before them. These represent the various human spirits which possess the sheikha during the ceremony. Then, recognizing the social status of group members, the main client has the place of honor after the sheikha, and those who have had Zar ceremonies previously in which blood was drawn from an animal or bird, i.e., the women have "killed," sit in chairs or double mats. Others who have "killed" but appear to be less important relations and friends, sit on benches or single mats. The rest sit on the ground. Social status is linked to Zar experiences; however it is women from higher socio-economic levels who can afford an elaborate Zar including "killing," so the systems overlap. It should be noted that the women who have "killed" may become assistants to the sheikha at other Zar ceremonies, thus enhancing their social status further. The sheikha always has the primary place of importance.

Additional planning includes providing accessories demanded by the sheikha. These may include a variety of sticks made from different materials and gathered from different parts of Sudan; fly switches, purses made of leather, amulets containing phrases from the Koran, beads from Europe and Africa and prayer beads, cigarettes and ash trays, incense bowls and coffee jebanas; old hats, including tajirs (Muslim skull caps), men's clothing, candles and rings; dresses in the colors associated with spirits. These are used at various times in the ceremony as the spirit moves the sheikha or clients.

(2) Individual and group discussions. The social nature of Zar makes discussion of problems easy among the women. While they wait for the ceremony to begin and during breaks in the ceremony, they talk among themselves. And even when the sheikha speaks alone to the client, she has probably already been informed by other women what is troubling the client. There are not many secrets. However, when a client speaks directly to the sheikha, who is supposedly providing her body as a vehicle for the spirit, the client feels she is safe from gossip because the sheikha supposedly has no knowledge of the conversation. So even her friends do not necessarily hear all aspects of her problems.

The frequency of Zar meetings, especially the regular Wednesday and Saturday meetings, permits women to talk and share experiences as they wait for the sheikha. There is thus continuity of sharing and providing group support.

(3) Specific actions. For the less formal Zar meetings, the following is rather typical of the actions taken. The recipient of the blessing is brought into a room with the sheikha and, after a formal greeting, is seated before the sheikha. The ceremony begins by pressing a bowl of burning incense against the top of the head, the shoulders and along the spine. The arms are then partly raised and the incense bowl run along their undersides. A similar performance then occurs with the legs, followed by holding both the hands and feet above the incense bowl and the joints of the fingers and toes are manipulated so that they crack. A newcomer writes down her most important wishes for the future, crumples the paper over the incense burner and deposits the slip inside a tambour (stringed musical instrument). Finally, a small group of the recipients of the blessing stand together while the sheikha beats a series of drums and tunelessly plucks the strings of the tambour. With this the Zar ends.

A more elaborate series of specific actions taken for other Zar ceremonies, when client complaints are more serious or the sheikha needs more powers to remove the offending spirit, involve the following actions. First, the sheikha may have to use her divination powers to diagnose cases of spirit possession by reading patterns formed by shells thrown on the ground and by interpreting dreams. The women at the Zar have made themselves more in tune with the spirits attending the ceremony by shaking each flagpole and rattling the shakers as they enter the place of the ceremony. The group ceremony begins with music provided by several drummers, with the sheikha as chief drummer. They begin to establish a simple, insistent rhythm, which after about 5 or 10 minutes stimulates some of the women to get up and dance. The music and dancing begin in quite a restrained fashion and build to a more frantic tempo, with the women hyperventilating as they dance. After dancing for 10 to 15 minutes, the women slump to the floor and look dazed and confused while there is a break in the drumming. Some women do not dance, but move their shoulders while sitting and hyperventilating.

Along with drumming are songs, including a special one for each of the 6 spirits associated with Zar. During the song of any particular spirit, only the women who have sacrificed a lamb to that spirit may dance standing up. The others must dance sitting or kneeling. Just a minority dance at any one time. Most merely sit and watch.

In addition to a song for each spirit is a drum beat for each spirit. The sheikha sometimes intones the names of the spirits using the different beat for each one and begins the intoning with the most powerful spirit. If she considers it necessary, the invoking of the spirit may require special dressing up to impersonate it, sometimes using the sticks, spears, cigarettes, special tobes and dresses or even men's clothing.

The common ritual pattern for these Zar is drumming, dancing, circulating the incense, and intervals of rest and smoking.

Finally, if spirits do not fully reveal their intentions, there is another ceremony called faith el elbe (opening of the box) which compels them to do so. The client inhales incense while the sheikha requests the spirits to reveal themselves and their demands. The client then drinks the blood of 2 doves specially slaughtered for the occasion, or has a lamb killed for the occasion, and is marked with the blood by the sheikha as an anointment.

The spirits usually ask for gifts in addition to the music and dancing and incense to appease them. The gifts are given to the client and are paid for by the husband.

d. Results. Satisfactory results are of two kinds. One is an elimination of the problem – the woman becomes pregnant, the husband does not take another wife, the pains or depression go away. The other is learning to live with the problem and controlling its more destructive aspects. This is aided by continuous attendance at Zar ceremonies as a spectator-participant or periodically as a major client. The group, aware of the status of each woman as far as Zar experiences and results are concerned, continues to act as a support system.

CONCLUSIONS

Zar as practiced among Sudanese women is an effective device for alleviating mental health problems and enhancing the social status of participants. The male domination of Sudanese cultures makes women vulnerable to arbitrary and capricious behavior on the part of men and limits women's rights to use the broader social, economic, religious, and political systems to address their grievances or to help shape policies that affect their lives. Women are generally regarded as weak, submissive creatures, while husbands are strong and may do as they wish. There are constant problems in polygamous marriages; divorce is easily obtained by men with even infertility being sufficient grounds. According to Cloudsley, "consciously or unconsciously, women employ Zar possession as a way of insinuating their interests and demands in the face of male constraint" (1983, p. 80).

Zar is particularly effective as it incorporates the universal concepts and assumptions in most successful treatments of mental health problems. It has adapted over the years to the unique needs of Sudanese women, or, perhaps more accurately, to the acceptable ways for addressing mental health problems in Sudanese society. There is every evidence that Zar will continue to make contributions to the well-being of Sudanese women over the years.

REFERENCES

Cris Ayton. (1984) The many faces of Zar. *Sudanow*, August, 41-43.

E. Cerilli. Zar (1983) *Encyclopedia of Islam-leiden*, 15, 1217.

Anne Cloudsley (1983) *Women of Omdurman*. London: Ethnographica.

Ncmat-Mubarak (1985) *Al-Zaar* Senior research paper, Ahfad University College for Women, Omdurman, Sudan.

Samia el Hadi el Nagar (1978) *Sudanow*, January, 38-40.

Women and AIDS

Ntiense Ben Edemikpong

INTRODUCTION

The question of where the AIDS virus originated is a matter of intense international debate. Some say that AIDS may have appeared first among the green monkeys of central Africa or perhaps in some backwater village in the interior of the continent. Two respected British scientists have even speculated that it could have been borne from outer space on a comet and washed to earth in rainfall (Lagos Weekend Newspaper, 1987). But Dr. Jonathan Mann, AIDS coordinator for the Geneva-based World Health Organization (WHO) said, "we believe there is no good evidence yet on where the virus came from, for the epidemic of clinical AIDS in Africa coincided in time with its appearance in Haiti, the USA and other countries" (Lagos Weekend Newspaper, 1987). Wherever the virus came from, one indisputable fact is that the terrifying scourge of AIDS is here and is spreading everywhere. Seldom has a single disease put so many people around the world at such great risk. The AIDS virus comes in a variety of strains and has the ability to mutate rapidly, making the development of potential vaccine highly problematic. It is an infection that seems to begin with few

Ntiense Ben Edemikpong was born at Ede Obuk-Eket in Akwa Ibom State of Nigeria on 11th November 1948, and was educated in the University of Ibadan-Nigeria where she obtained the Diploma in Religious Studies and Philosophy in 1977; and graduated in the Ecumenical Institute of Seminary Studies, Norwalk, California, USA with the B. Th. (Bachelor of Theology) in 1980. She has been a strong advocate of Women's rights and joined the Women's Centre-Eket as a patron in 1982. She has since then been the Director of Research and Organization of The Women's Centre and the author of articles of The Women's Centre such as "We shall not fold our Arms and wait — Female Genital Mutilation," "Monkey do work. Baboon de chop."

or no symptoms yet many develop into a full scale lethal form. The so-called AIDS-Related complex (ARC), frequently a pre-cursor of AIDS, is a disease syndrome that can be deadly in itself. And doctors believe that some people who have been exposed to the virus (known as seropositives) may never develop AIDS, though they may still be infectious to others.

AFRICAN NATIONS AND AIDS POLITICS

According to a report released in June 1987 by the World Health Organization (WHO), about 50,000,000 Africans were supposed to be carrying AIDS and the disease had reached epidemic proportions in Central, East and Southern Africa. Many African nations are often outraged and embarrassed when their countries are associated with AIDS and have sometimes refused to cooperate with women's groups and organizations that make such revelations to Western sources. Zambia, for instance, has banned health authorities and women's organizations from sending any information on AIDS outside the country and even when the son of the Zambian president died of AIDS, it was not made public until a year later. Zimbabwe has refused to assist with funding the projects or programs of all women's organizations that release the latest figures of AIDS carriers in the country to the outside world. Kenya, with 10,000 cases of AIDS, has so far continued to deny the existence of that magnitude of AIDS and has blamed the Western media for gross exaggeration of figures. At the International AIDS conference held in June 1987 in Washington, DC, a revelation was made by Dr. Robert Gallo, an American AIDS specialist, that 10 Nigerians were identified with a special AIDS virus which he termed the "Nigerian Red Virus." In the usual reaction of African governments over the association of AIDS with their countries, the leader of the Nigerian delegation at the conference, Dr. E. Essien became outraged with Dr. Gallo's revelation and emphatically denied the existence of the "Nigerian Red Virus." The government of Uganda, which seems to have the greatest share of people with AIDS in Africa, has opined that it sees no point in making people panic when there is no risk of an epidemic. Thus African nations for political, economic and social reasons continue to deny the threat of this disease to the citizens of their countries. Nonetheless, many European and Asian countries have imposed questionable and xenophobic restrictions on people of African descent, thereby prompting a scrambling to hide or distort numbers of people with AIDS. Kenya is now suffering from decreased tourism because of unrestrained announcement of its AIDS cases, says Dr. Bassey Edem, a medical doctor in Uye (capital of Akwa Ibom State of Nigeria) about the distortion of AIDS figures in Africa. He stated: "ultimately we will all suffer from hasty and panic measures. It is humanity that will bear the brunt of these distortions. I am convinced more people have AIDS than are being reported" (Edem, 1988).

POSSIBLE EFFECTS AND MOVES FOR COMBAT

The refugee, famine and drought problems in Africa today are not of more threat to human lives than is AIDS, yet while the battle to fight AIDS is raging in Western countries African nations are daily denying the threat of AIDS to their citizens so that their so-called national image abroad may not be tarnished. An Italian source has revealed that an average person with AIDS incurs hospital bills of roughly $110,000 which could potentially bankrupt a country's public health system if the number surges. Will the national economies of the already impoverished African countries that develop a carefree attitude to the existence of AIDS in their countries not be in jeopardy? The USA budgetary allocation to AIDS has risen from $5.5 million to $450 million in the past 5 years. Britain has unleashed a media campaign to alert and enlighten the public on the killer disease. The Italian health ministry is spending $40 million to set up treatment centers. The anxiety is much the same throughout Europe and the U.S. but in Africa, the response has not by the least fraction matched the problem. Are countries, especially the poorer ones, in danger of allocating resources to AIDS control more under the influence of media exaggeration and external pressure than cool appraisal of the cost of the benefits? In almost every country there is intense debate between those who answer "yes," and those who believe that while AIDS prevention may exact costs today, these are small in comparison to the penalties which increased HIV infection could inflict tomorrow. Costa Rica provides a clear example of this calculus. It has achieved a five-fold decrease in child mortality to 18 per 1000 over a 30 year period up to 1986. Tunisia and the Congo with almost the same per capita spending on health, have child mortality rates of 74 and 75 per 1000. One reason for the difference has been Costa Rica's determined emphasis on primary health, coupled with its comprehensive social insurance system. But the success is threatened by AIDS. Despite the fact that, internationally, AIDS has meant increased funding for certain activities in the health sector, it is undeniable that the HIV epidemic is drawing resources away from other vital areas of disease prevention and health promotion. At the very least, experienced researchers, doctors, nurses, technicians and health planners are finding that AIDS is increasingly diverting their attention and energy away from other urgent problems. Caribbean, Ugandan, Haitian, Kenyan, Rwandan, Zairean and other health workers relate similar experiences of priorities turned upside down by AIDS. And the USA authorities point out that a recent resurgence of syphilis is probably due to the fact that it has been neglected while the focus has switched to AIDS (U.S. Centers for Disease Control, 1988).

AIDS AND CIRCUMCISION

In addition, it is the sexual aspects of AIDS that have riveted public attention on the disease and this is not without good cause. Sexual transmission is the most common route of contracting AIDS. Some 55 to 75 percent of AIDS in Europe and the U.S. have occurred in homosexual men between the ages of 20 to 40 years and among intravenous drug users who share dirty hypodermic needles. But the opposite is the case in Africa where unprotected heterosexual intercourse is the cause of the present widespread transmission of AIDS. Recent research findings have also attributed the transmission of AIDS in Africa to cultural factors and one of these is the practice of female genital mutilation. Uli Linke, an anthropologist and researcher in Toronto had this to say about her recent research (1986): "I noticed a prevailing assumption that the same cultural factors were at work in the transmission of AIDS in Africa as those in Europe and the USA — namely sexual promiscuity, the use of unclean hypodermic needles and homosexuality. None of these points explain the equal ratio of men and women contracting the disease in Central Africa. The bottom line in the transmission of AIDS is the exchange of the body fluids particularly blood, which gave me the idea that it might be related to female circumcision." Linke stated: "the most extreme form of female circumcision in Africa, infibulation is the complete removal of the vulval tissue including the clitoris and the labia. After the tissue had been removed the sides of the wound are often sewn together leaving a miniscule opening perhaps the size of a matchstick. No anesthetic is used in the operation which lasts between 15 to 20 minutes and the instruments used are not sterilized. Essentially sexual intercourse is then impossible unless in some form or another the vagina is reopened. This is usually accomplished through forcible entry by the husband which often leads to hemorrhaging." In women, Linke writes, "infibulation is associated not only with chronic pain, but with lesions in the vaginal tissue and bleeding leading to the presence of blood during intercourse. In some cases full penetration can take up to nine months during which time anal intercourse is a common alternative." In a letter to the professional journal *Science* in January 1986, Linke stressed that, "it is noteworthy that the recent outbreak of AIDS in Africa corresponds geographically to those regions in which female genital mutilation is still practiced."

Fran Hosken, another researcher on female genital mutilation, has written: "in many Muslim areas of Africa girls are married at a very young age to much older men who can afford to pay the steep bride price. The genitalia of these girls are often very small and are closed by infibulation; tradition therefore demands that the husband must have prolonged sex in the wedding night and that blood must flow in the genitals to confirm the brides' virginity. Thus the girl-brides are torn by the much larger males during intercourse. As a result of this operation, as well as other sexual practices by men that involve lacerations and the flow of blood in the female genital area, AIDS has many opportunities to reach women who are infected during sexual intercourse" (Hosken, 1987, p. 45).

In addition, a survey conducted recently by the Women's Centre, Eket in Nigeria has authenticated the above research revelations. The survey was conducted in two African Countries, Uganda and Equatorial Guinea. Of the 172 pregnant women tested whether they had AIDS-virus antibodies in Uganda, 129 proved positive and out of this number, 86 were those whose genitalia were mutilated. In Equatorial Guinea, of the 100 women tested, 78 proved positive and out of this number, 65 were those whose genitalia were mutilated (Women's Centre, Eket, 1987). Indeed, medical authorities tell us that sexual lifestyles which injure the body and cause mixing of blood play a role in the transmission of retroviruses such as AIDS (as does sharing intravenous needles) (Glocce, 1988). Therefore, the practice whereby a newly married man must have prolonged sex in the wedding night with an infibulated girl bride so that blood must flow in the genital area to confirm the girl's virginity puts them at high risk for AIDS infection. In further consideration of Professor Linke's revelation it is apparent that a genitally mutilated woman is exposed to double risks from AIDS infection; for where a husband cannot gain a full penetration of his wife during sexual intercourse, anal intercourse may be a common alternative. According to Dr. M. Paalman, Director of the Netherlands Foundation for STD control, "anal intercourse carries the highest risk for infection of all sexual techniques. Therefore it is better to refrain from it entirely" (Paalman 1988, p. 15).

Although Dr. Elizabeth Reid, consultant with the Health Advancement Division in the Australian Department of Health, has asserted that "a number of social customs relating to women must now be reconsidered for AIDS risk factors. One of these is the use of the blade or other instrument in female circumcision. There is no evidence as yet by this means, but the practice puts women potentially at risk" (Reid, 1988, p. 29). The Women's Centre in Eket, Nigeria has strongly rejected the latter part of Dr. Reid's assertion that "there is no evidence as yet by this means. . . ." In many parts of Africa genital mutilation is performed by traditional circumcisors or traditional birth attendants who charge a fee for the operation. The knives or blades used for the operation are rarely sterilized and are often infected with the samples of blood of past victims. On a circumcision day all girls for the operation are gathered in the family compound and five to ten girls can be mutilated at a stretch with a single blood-stained unsterilized knife or blade. This provides an opportunity therefore for each victim to share blood. Moreover, female circumcision, as Dr. Reid has asserted, is a misleading term used to describe all kinds of mutilation. Included under this term is circumcision, which is the cutting of the prepuce of the vagina and is the mildest form of mutilation. Also included under the term circumcision is excision, which is the cutting of the clitoris and of all or part of the labia minora; the worst of it all is infibulation which is the cutting of the clitoris, labia minora and at least the anterior two thirds and often the whole of the medial part of the majora. The two sides are stitched together except for a small opening left for the passage of urine or menstrual blood. One must therefore wonder which of these three mutilations she was referring to. From our standpoint we have attested to the fact that female genital mutilation increases the widespread transmission of AIDS in Africa.

OTHER FACTORS

In Africa, which is a patriarchal society, the man is the owner of all material goods produced within the family. Polygamy, which is a system whereby a man possesses a number of wives, is a common practice. Under this custom, a man is required to pay a bride price for marriage to a young girl and in many cases these so-called husbands are old enough to be grandfathers of these brides. In many societies it is common for a man to marry four to six wives. Thus each man has multiple sexual partners. If the husband of six wives is infested with AIDS, the wives are placed at a high risk of infection. Moreover, African traditional religions and Islam encourage and endorse polygamy. Islam, for instance, permits its adherents to marry up to four wives. Even when women are aware of the risk of transmission, they may find it difficult to insist on protected sexual intercourse because of their subordinate position in society in which they are regarded as appendages to their husbands. Inadequate care by the husbands, complications during childbirth, pregnancies occurring too close together, undernourishment, anemia, and other biological burdens place women's bodies at risk for AIDS to thrive; therefore the offspring of these women succumb readily to AIDS and diarrheal diseases. The adverse effects on the health of mother and child of pregnancies occurring too close together or in teenaged mothers and women over age 35 are also well known. When the age at marriage is low and childbearing starts early, many women become grandmothers in their forties. In high-mortality countries the likelihood of a woman being widowed after the age of 50 is high. Maternal deaths due to complications during labor and childbirth are over 100 times greater than in the developed world, and with women at immediate risk of death, avoidance of blood transfusion is impossible. The principle of voluntary blood donation is upheld more or less throughout Africa, but smaller blood banks rely on relatives of patients. Relatives may recruit and pay donors without the knowledge of the donor panel organizers. In most cases this blood is not screened due to lack of AIDS screening equipment and even where there may be equipment those trained to use them may not be available. Recently, it has been revealed that at the University of Calabar Teaching Hospital in Nigeria there was equipment for screening blood meant for transfusion but unscreened blood was still used in transfusion. When the Medical Director of the Hospital was contacted about this issue, he complained of lack of trained staff to operate the equipment for clinical analysis. The few staff members who could operate the equipment were only using it for research purposes. In urban central Africa, seropositivity for HIV infection was found in 18% of blood donors tested in Kigali (Rwanda), 14% in Bukoba, 4.4% in Dar-es-Salaam (Tanzania), 10% in Brazzaville (Congo), and 18.4% in Lusaka (Zambia) (Fleming, 1988). These facts strongly implicate blood transfusion in the transmission of HIV to women suffering from maternal complications.

A CHANCE TO SPEAK OUT

Given the fatal nature of AIDS and its possible association with female genital mutilation, multiple sexual partners, polygamy, and blood transfusion, women cannot afford to take chances. Women must have the opportunities to have a say in matters that affect their lives or the lives of their children. This can be brought about to a large extent through education, which has been recognized all over the world as a great agent of change. While the feverish quest for a treatment or a vaccine for AIDS continues, health education is now the only main tool we have with which to counter this disease and women especially at the grassroots level must be made aware of how the virus is transmitted and how it is not transmitted. AIDS prevention and control strategies can be implemented effectively and efficiently, and can be evaluated in a manner that respects and protects human rights. The women should be informed that there is no public health rationale to justify isolation or any discriminatory measures based solely on the fact that a person is known to be HIV infected. They must be told that transmission and HIV spreads entirely through identifiable behaviors and specific actions which are subject to individual control.

Meanwhile, AIDS discrimination is occurring in many African countries. Telling a patient that he or she has HIV is a difficult decision for Tanzanian doctors, says a military officer who was unaware early this year that he had AIDS (Ogola, 1989), "when I requested drinking water I was told to fetch it. When I asked for a cup the nurse left but never returned." As his health deteriorated, his wife, relatives and friends suspecting he might have AIDS, stopped coming to see him. The avoidance of discrimination against persons suspected to be HIV infected is important for AIDS prevention and control; failure to prevent such discrimination may endanger public health. Women's organizations have an important role to play in this regard. They have the potential to assume a direct preventive role and a means of reaching not only into each village and community but into each household, and providing information and education to persons with behaviors that place them at the risk of HIV infection and exposure to HIV infected persons. They can also counsel HIV infected persons and ensure the safety of blood and other invasive practices and procedures. In Nigeria, for instance, the Women's Centre in Eket has launched a massive education campaign by visiting homes, touring the countryside, providing newspaper, radio and television information about AIDS, and educating about the negative effects of female genital mutilation and other traditional practices that endanger the lives of women. In India, women have organized themselves against rape and in Kenya against men who are under the influence of alcoholism. The education of women by women can be expected to bring an immediate change in women's beliefs, practices and the relationship between women and men, and at the same time give women greater independence from men.

REFERENCES

Edem, B. (1988). Anton Clinic, Uyo-Nigeria, Personal Communication.

Fleming, A. F. (March 1988). Global impact of AIDS. Conference, London School of Hygiene and Tropical Medicine, London, England.

Glocce, E. (1988). AIDS—A Medical Bonanza. *Nexus New Times*.

Hosken, F. (1987). Female Circumcision. *Win News* P. 46.

Linke, U. (1986). Personal Communication, Anthropology Dept. University of California. Berkeley, California.

Lagos Weekend Newspaper (Jan. 23, 1987). AIDS—The Fear Spreads, P. 3.

Ogola, H. (January, 1989). World AIDS, London, England.

Paalman, M. (November, 1988). Safer Sex. *World Health Magazine*, WHO. Geneva, Switzerland.

Reid, E. (March, 1988). Women and AIDS. *World Health Magazine*, WHO. Geneva, Switzerland.

U.S. Centers for Disease Control. (1988). *Morbidity and Mortality Weekly*, Special Report, P. 3.

Women's Centre, Eket Nigeria (1987). Unpublished Manuscript, Vol. 1.

AIDS in Uganda as a Gender Issue

Mere Nakateregga Kisekka

INTRODUCTION

Uganda, a beautiful landlocked East African nation of 15.4 million people, was, up to the early seventies, a tourist haven. Since 1974, however, it attracted international headlines more for negative happenings than anything else. Over the past decade, Uganda has been saddled with the bloody military rule of dictator Idi Amin followed by civil strife and guerrilla war that have destroyed much of the country's social, economic and political fabric. The AIDS epidemic is the latest in the series of scourges that have hit the nation.

This article is based on information gathered through visits to Uganda between 1981 and the end of 1988 by the author. The author herself, a Ugandan with family and friends residing in the most AIDS-affected district in the country, was able to gather qualitative data from informal interviews with relatives of people with AIDS and relevant categories of the public such as youths, elders and health professionals. In addition, non-academic sources such as

The author is a Ugandan lecturer engaged in teaching and research in Nigeria since 1974, in the areas of medical sociology, social psychology and women's studies. She is a past Vice President of the Association of African Women for Research and Development (1983-1988) and the current national coordinator of the Women's Health Network in Nigeria.

This article is a revised version of a paper titled "Sexually Transmitted Diseases as a Gender issue: Examples from Nigeria and Uganda" by M.N. Kisekka and B.N. Otesanya presented at the Association of African Women for Research and Development Seminar and General Assembly Meeting, 8-14 August, 1988, Dakar, Senegal.

Requests for reprints may be sent to Dr. Mere Kisekka, Dept. Sociology, Ahmadu Bello University, Zaria, Nigeria.

35

daily newspapers, popular magazines, television and radio features were utilized.

THE OFFICIAL VIEW: PREVALENCE

In Uganda, AIDS is referred to as SLIM due to the extreme weight loss. According to a Kenyan source (the Weekly Review, February 17, 1989) a Kenyan researcher, Dr. G.S. Gashibi, quoted an August 1988 survey of the cumulative rates of AIDS cases per 100,000 which named Uganda as the third highest African country with AIDS, and seventh in the world with a ratio of 25.82 cases. Specifically, the Uganda Ministry of Health recorded 5664 AIDS cases (Republic of Uganda, 1988). Of the 5455 cases (96%) that had gender specified, 2641 (48%) of them were male and 2814 (52.%) were female. Of the 3711 AIDS cases whose location of health care at the time of diagnosis could be identified, 70% were inpatients and 30% were outpatients. With respect to age, there were 519 cases under five years which indicated the equally important perinatal and childbirth routes of transmission. For females, the age group most represented was 20-24 with 800 cases, while the corresponding age peak for males was 25-29 with 500 cases. The spread of AIDS is such that 32 of the 33 districts in the country have been affected, with Kampala (35%) and Masaka (23%) reporting the highest number.

In an interview with Dr. Okware, the Director of AIDS control program in Uganda, he stressed that the disease was transmitted largely through heterosexual relations. He based his assertion on studies carried out in the country which revealed that on samples of 135 individuals there was no infection among pre-puberty children aged 5 to 14 years, nor among adults aged 60 years and over. On the contrary, 85% of the infected men were in the 15-39 age group, and 14% in the 40-54 age category. Similarly, Dr. Okware reported that in a survey of 114 household contacts of 25 homes in which a member of the household had AIDS, only sexual partners were found to be infected. This finding was cited as evidence to dispel the notion that AIDS can be contracted through casual social interaction.

THE OFFICIAL VIEW: ORIGIN

Regarding the origin of AIDS, the Ministry of Health of Uganda is emphatic that the first AIDS case was identified in 1983 at Kasensero village in the Rakai district, two years after AIDS had been recognized (June, 1981) in the United States and central Africa. Hooper (1987) reports that Kasensero village is situated on the shores of Lake Victoria and it consists primarily of fishermen, people dealing in the black market, and barmaids; about 200 people who constitute a quarter of its population are reported to have so far perished with AIDS.

THE OFFICIAL VIEW: CONTROL

In terms of infrastructural facilities, Uganda is ill-equipped to deal with the AIDS epidemic. The existing 81 hospitals (28 non-governmental), 89 health centers, 94 maternity centers, and 463 dispensaries or aid posts (Republic of Uganda, 1988) are grossly inadequate in terms of drugs, facilities and personnel.

This bleak situation is, however, redeemed by the bold step of the country's leadership in acknowledging and publicizing the magnitude of the AIDS epidemic and launching a well-orchestrated and vigorous five-year AIDS program which includes educational, medical and epidemiological surveillance measures to counter the situation.

For the time being the government is not enthusiastic about (neither does it have the capacity for) compulsory blood screening for HIV infection because of the well-founded fear that disclosure of positive results might lead to desperate or vengeful acts. Therefore, blood screening is limited to purposes of diagnosis and blood transfusion. At Mulago (government) hospitals in Kampala and Masaka, people with AIDS are isolated in special male and female wards and pregnant women with AIDS deliver in isolated labor rooms.

The government has mobilized the resources and channels of the private and public mass media, the entertainment sector through songs and plays, and the church, in its public AIDS awareness campaign. The recurrent message is "zero grazing," meaning sexual fidelity is depicted on television and radio (in Uganda there is an

estimated ownership of 0.3 million T.V. sets and 3 million radios)
and also printed in the newspapers (estimated literacy is 50% of the
population).

It is remarkable that there is a virtual absence of moral condem-
nation by all these sources including religious institutions. Thus,
the country's Catholic Medical Bureau enjoins *tobaliga* ("love
faithfully") and stresses the message of compassion rather than
judgment with reference to Luke 6, 36-37. Similarly the Protestant
Medical Bureau emphasizes that "AIDS is deadly" and preaches
monogamy in marriage while calling on Christians to treat people
with AIDS according to Matthew (25: 31-46) with food, drink,
clothing, shelter, nursing care and comfort. These same messages
are delivered in the pulpits, and there is hardly a church sermon
which does not call for prayers for people with AIDS. Similarly,
children who are orphans or either one of whose parents died of
AIDS, are authorized to receive aid (e.g., bedding, clothes, tinned
foods, etc.) donated by international relief agencies to victims of
the countries's protracted reign of terror and successive wars of
liberation.

Among the government's far-reaching educational measures are:
(1) production of numerous brochures and posters in English and
major local languages which are posted in health facilities, government offices, bus stations, and other public gathering places; (2)
training of trainers identified as modern and traditional health workers, parents and teachers, religious and women's organizations and
political bodies. These groups are educated through seminars and
regular in-service training; and (3) special campaigns which are tar-
geted at groups at high risk for AIDS, such as prostitutes and their
customers in bars and hotels. Among youths, the campaign focuses
on the school population since 60% of all Ugandan children aged 6-
13 years and approximately 10% of all adolescents aged 14-19
years attend schools (Republic of Uganda Ministry of Health 1988).
Characteristically, adolescent and adult women of fertile age are
singled out as bearers of morality. African society characteristically
focuses on women for problems of sexuality and fertility. Thus,
women are perceived as the sources of sexually transmitted diseases
and therefore the custodians of morality. Likewise, in its educational campaign, the government focuses on women to receive mes-

sages enjoining them to adhere "to a strict monogamous behavior and to require the same from husbands or sexual partners."

It is against this background of the official AIDS situation in the country that we must now proceed to examine the populace's attitudinal and behavioral configurations with regards to the AIDS phenomenon.

PUBLIC PERCEPTION OF AND BEHAVIORS TOWARDS AIDS AND ITS VICTIMS

The Ugandan public perceives AIDS with a mixture of natural and supernatural orientations. On the naturalistic level, there is widespread acceptance of sexual transmission as a major route of AIDS. In this regard it is believed that Tanzanian soldiers spread the disease during the invasion that overthrew dictator Idi Amin in 1979. There is also the fear of its being contagious, although this is a development of the late eighties.

From the supernaturalistic angle, there is a belief that Ugandans who used to conduct trading expeditions to Tanzania cheated their customers. Consequently a certain Tanzanian tribe known as *Bakerebwe* and reputed for skills in witchcraft, is alleged to have retaliated by casting spells in the form of AIDS. Therefore AIDS is regarded as a measure of distributive justice on Ugandans who partook in any of the smuggled Tanzanian goods, whether knowingly or unknowingly. In this respect, AIDS is *omuteego* or randomly selecting its victims.

Epidemiologically, there is a consensus that AIDS is one disease which has affected people of varying social categories but particularly *abatambuze*, the "promiscuous" ones. Also, the youth or *abavubuka* are regarded as prominently at risk.

News of an AIDS death of a prominent personality such as a doctor, lawyer, entertainer, or business person travels fast and wide and raises concern, speculations of insecurity, and speculations about the fate of the deceased's sexual contacts over the years. Gossip and rumors start circulating about potential sexual contacts of the deceased.

In the villages near Kalisizo town where the researcher conducted her investigation, many households in which one or more people died of AIDS were cited. Some individuals at various stages of infection, with one or more of the related AIDS complex symptoms, were seen sitting or lying down on the veranda being greeted by passers-by. The fact that in some of these households a parent as well as his/her grown-up offspring has died of AIDS sustains the myth of supernaturalistic causation of AIDS on the one hand, and the myth of casual contagion on the other.

In the early years of AIDS in Uganda, when its etiology was unknown, people who had AIDS were regarded with pity. Progressively however, the overriding response is characterized by avoidance as displayed in reluctance to shake hands, share dishes or come in close physical contact with anyone suspected of having AIDS. Thus in bars and restaurants, customers have formed a habit of drinking beer out of straws. Correspondingly, the (Anglican) Church of Uganda had to yield to social pressure by discontinuing the practice of sharing holy communion from a common chalice.

Likewise, in public transportation, people either force out a person suspected of having AIDS or vacate the premise as a precautionary measure. These discriminatory behaviors have extended to funeral ceremonies whereby a person who has died of AIDS is hurriedly buried without observing all traditional protocols or sharing his/her personal effects.

Perhaps the most drastic reaction to the AIDS situation was highlighted in the Taifa Empya newspaper (Aug 19, 1987) in which Masaka town residents were reported as suggesting that as an epidemiological measure, the government should quarantine women related to people with AIDS, while men should be castrated!

Furthermore, individuals (especially young women) of slim physical statures are particularly stereotyped as having AIDS. Men, therefore, feel more secure with plump girls for casual sexual companionship. But that line of defense has been gradually broken these days, as one hears quick reminders and retorts about fat people only offering short-lived security as they might in fact be in the asymptomatic stages of AIDS.

It is a measure of the prevalence of AIDS in Uganda that it has become a daily topic of conversation around which jokes, riddles, abuses, sarcasm and crude invectives are woven. Even pre-school children can be heard in their play threatening to infect one another with AIDS. Every ailment and death is feared and/or rumored to be AIDS-related. It is remarkable that in every encounter with an individual or group of individuals that the researcher made, one of the first questions that she was consistently asked concerned whether AIDS was also a problem in Nigeria, her country of residence; the fact that this was a spontaneous reaction that occurred without the researcher's direct or indirect prompting, clearly demonstrates people's anxiety to ascertain their comparative level of confrontation with the AIDS epidemic.

Business-wise, the informal sector has been drastically hit by the AIDS epidemic. Lodging and rooming houses which sprang up in many towns and trading centers in the early eighties to cater to travelers and disco-party goers who wanted quick or overnight sexual liaisons, have undergone decline in patronage. In the same manner, food vendors specializing in freshly-squeezed juices of orange, passion fruit or banana wine are experiencing low returns, as people fear contamination of AIDS from these home-made drinks.

But, as expected, the most devastating consequences are on the individuals with AIDS, and their immediate circle of family and friends. The certainty of an agonizing and undignifying death has caused revulsion and despair. Moreover, most people experience residual bitterness and anguish over what appears to them as an irrational and random selection of attack. This feeling of frustration and victimization has often elicited responses of intrapunitive and extrapunitive aggression. To this end, many instances of suicides by poisoning with insecticides have been reported. Vengeful acts attributed to people with AIDS are widely rumored as well. These include rape, concerted efforts to sexually entice as many women as possible with money, and urination and defecation in public streams and wells. Other people with AIDS or relatives of people who have died of AIDS, migrate from their localities to distant places where they are anonymous. Prostitutes have salvaged their livelihood by impersonating school girls and thus escaping the stereotype of a high risk group. The public therefore seems justified in its perception that people with AIDS tend to revenge (*sifa bwomu*) by recklessly seeking sexual contacts with unsuspecting strangers.

Inevitably, unsettling implications of the AIDS epidemic on sexuality and nuptiality have also arisen. There is a pervasive morbid feeling of fatalism or pessimism expressed, especially among single people, to the effect that every eligible person is a potential source of contracting AIDS. Young people hesitate to get married as they fear that eligible people might already have been infected with the AIDS virus. Also, those who are already overseas for studies or career training tend to prolong their stay because of uncertainty of the health statuses of future partners at home. In other circles, sex, whether with a spouse or a friend, has become tinted with fear of AIDS as there is always a lingering mutual suspicion of an occasional current or even past sexual contact with someone at risk for AIDS.

Many people have come to regard AIDS as a panacea for the male double sex standard. Yet others, men in particular, have redefined "safe sex" to include extramarital affairs with a married person. Thus they are unwilling to cultivate monogamy.

IMPACT ON HEALTH SEEKING AND DELIVERY

One of the most visible adverse effects of Uganda's last fifteen years of political and economic turmoil was the virtual collapse of the health delivery system. This situation prompted the growth and proliferation of numerous privately-owned clinics, maternity wards, pharmacies, and itinerant druggists and "injection men." Interestingly, the itinerant groups invariably consisted of employees or ex-employees from hospitals or veterinary posts. In these institutions they were employed as orderlies, clerks, and assistants; due to their experiences and access to drugs, they seize the opportunity to moonlight in health delivery in the informal sector.

Given the past and current devastated state of the economy, it is doubtful that even with the best of credentials, a significant number of private facilities could conceivably afford sustained utilization of sterilized instruments. Neither of course can the majority of patients afford these services, and therefore they continue to patronize the itinerant druggists and "injection men" who operate on market days and around the villages and towns. Yet the favored method of sterilization by these "injection men" is to prick the used needle in a banana stem. In light of these observations, it is probable that the private health delivery system has contributed to the high prevalence of AIDS in the country.

Secondly, there has emerged a number of self-proclaimed "experts" in the treatment of AIDS who vigorously advertise their services in the mass media. Two of the prominent experts are Dr. Rashid Lukwago of Lyantonde in Rakai district and Dr. Sebabi of Makerere University. Dr. Lukwago is a traditional medical doctor who claims cures for AIDS, cancer and other terminal diseases. Dr. Sebabi is said to be a biochemist or laboratory technician who has had strong confrontations with the nation's AIDS control program personnel concerning his claims. As of the time of this investigation he had publicized through the daily newspapers a cure of at least fifty people with AIDS. He asserted that AIDS manifests itself in seven stages and that if a person was treated during the first five stages, it was possible to arrest the progress of the disease and effect a cure. Ironically, he seems to be persuasive with a sizable proportion of the public, including the educated class, supporting him in his struggle with the AIDS control program. The view is that the AIDS Control Program personnel are envious of his discovery of the cure for AIDS and are therefore merely suppressing him. On their part, the AIDS control officials consider Dr. Sebabi a quack and an embarrassment to the scientific community, who unfortunately is complicating the misery of people with AIDS with his ineffective cures and exorbitant fees.

The AIDS epidemic has created intense anxiety which has been reflected both in health seeking and illness behaviors. With some people it has evoked a state of "healthism" (Crawford, 1980), that is, an undue concern with staying healthy. In this regard any ailment is feared as an AIDS opportunistic infection and therefore drives one in search of an immediate cure as a test of proof or disproof of infection. The result is self-medication and usually over-medication and therefore spending an inordinate proportion of one's earnings on the purchase of manufactured drugs.

The other extreme response is one of phobia of or refusal to come in contact with health personnel, facilities, and equipment on the suspicion of their being contaminated with AIDS. It is partly this phobia which is the basis of widely-held allegations that hospital staff utilize the same syringes and needles for many patients and that many of the nurses are HIV seropositive. Actually it was gathered that hospitals do not as a matter of policy dismiss workers with AIDS. For example, a female nurse with AIDS was observed at Mulago Hospital in Kampala going about her duties. The head-nurse explained that such infected nurses were restricted only from coming in direct contact with the patients and were allowed to continue work until they progressed to the level where they would be incapacitated in performing regular duties.

This shows how the health system is confronted with humanitarian, ethical and medical issues of unprecedented proportions. The workers are, for example, gripped with mounting anxiety of contracting AIDS from patients through accidental pricking with needles or contact with contaminated blood through other means. For example, a nurse-midwife who runs a maternity home located ten kilometres from Masaka town and who had just returned from a visit in Britain, explained that she was no longer prescribing injections and that she was contemplating closing down the maternity home as it was located in an AIDS epidemic area. Another private clinic in the area devised an elaborate method of retaining each disposable syringe and needle for each particular patient for the duration of treatment, for it was explained that disposables were discarded only after several usages due to financial constraints. Patients who can afford the cost preferred and were advised to buy their own syringes and needles whenever they visited any facility. An interview with a dentist revealed that he planned to reduce cases of tooth extraction and scaling as a protective measure against infection from patients. He also reported that since he could not afford to buy great quantities of hand gloves he economized by washing or sterilizing and then re-using them. This method could be ineffective if the gloves are of poor quality.

SEXUAL HARASSMENT

The proportion of women who contract AIDS through sexual aggression or harassment may never be known but certainly should not be glossed over. It is necessary to note that sexual harassment has been defined as a phenomenon of power struggle such that it is "usually initiated and negotiated by a person in a position of authority and is sustained at the expense of another who cannot counter demands without the risk of reprisal" (Brandenburg, 1982, p. 322). As such, it is emphasized that sexual harassment should be recognized as an exploitation of a power relationship rather than as an exclusively sexual issue. Within this general conceptual framework, incidents of rape, sexual child abuse, and incest constitute sexual harassment.

Case A: A man's continuation of sexual involvement after the death of a sexual partner due to AIDS.

Mukasa was married to two women (Rozi and Bess) who lived in separate villages. He was living with Rozi, the senior wife, on a more permanent basis when she developed AIDS and died after about one year of infection.

Mukasa then moved in with Bess, the junior wife. After about fourteen months, Bess's young teenage sister, who was living with them developed the symptoms of AIDS. In a panic, Bess quickly returned her to her parents where she died of AIDS after six months. Everybody suspected Mukasa to be the sexual contact.

A year later, Joy a young woman who had also had a brief affair with Mukasa, died. Several months afterwards Mukasa died, followed by the deaths of Bess and their one-year-old child. They have left several orphans. Several village men are in a panic as they had had sexual encounters with Joy.

Since traditionally widows do not remarry, whereas widowers are encouraged to remarry, husbands of women who have died of AIDS are likely to continue the menace of spreading AIDS to women as long as they do not practice safer sex.

Furthermore, in Uganda there is ample evidence that incessant military and guerrilla warfares have for the most part institutionalized brutalization of the populace including sexual harassment with a concomitant rise in sexually transmitted diseases (STDs), particularly AIDS. For example, the North of the country was free from AIDS until after the battleground shifted following President Museveni's victory in May, 1986. The high rate of AIDS among the soldiers, reportedly at the rate of one in three, combined with their habitual harassment of women, leaves no doubt of their role in the epidemiology of the disease.

The AIDS situation has triggered other unexpected acts of marital sexual violence. In some quarters, men who had been used to constant extra-marital sex and who are now monogamous with their wives were reported to be increasingly sexually violent with their wives as a result of their frustrations. On the other hand, other men are accusing their wives of provoking sexual aggression by refusing their husband's sexual advances because of fear that the husbands might have AIDS due to extra-marital sexual relations or as mere reprisals for husbands' past extra-marital relations. A case below from Kampala captures one aspect of AIDS-related aggression.

Case B: A husband's violence towards his wife.

Recently, on outskirts of the city centre, a husband allegedly assaulted his wife because she refused to have sex with him. She was fearful that his former philandering ways might have inflicted him with the disease.

For almost two years he had totally ignored her until now. But she wanted no part of him. His reaction was to viciously beat her up.

Few would condone such behavior. But, then again, as one sympathetic man noted on the incident: "she was his wife. He had every right to sleep with her if he so wished."

Perhaps this is a chauvinistic point of view, but it is important to note the husband's violent reaction is an example of the extreme consequences of zero-grazing. It can be exceedingly frustrating for those men not used to excessive domesticity. (Mulinde-Musoke 1987, p. 10)

It is noteworthy that overall, these acts of sexual harassment with actual or potential risk of spreading AIDS are invariably perpetrated by men against women.

REPRODUCTIVE RIGHTS

AIDS has touched a central issue on the topic of women's health, that is, reproductive health and associated rights. For example, women might be pregnant when they discover that they or their husbands have AIDS. This raises the issue of mandatory versus voluntary screening of pregnant women for the AIDS virus, and the right to abort in the instance of positive cases. In the village studied, there were several cases of babies born with the AIDS virus, many of whom did not survive long; they thus bear testimony to perinatal or postnatal route of AIDS transmission.

Taking cognizance of the human and particularly the African desire to immortalize oneself, it is probable that some infected individuals may strive to reproduce in order to leave a survivor after their own imminent deaths. Certainly, all these issues raise complex legal and ethical factors for Ugandan women which can only be solved or at least reduced by a concerted program of counseling and related policy measures.

Of equal relevance to women's reproductive rights is the controversy regarding the relationship between breast-feeding and transmission of the AIDS virus to suckling babies. It must be realized that whether the evidence is conclusive or not, the mere publicity of the debate will probably deter some high-risk mothers from breast-feeding. If this happens, it is feared to culminate in more cases of infant mortality due to malnutrition and decreased immunology to infant diseases. This then is potentially an endless vicious cycle, with more childbearing, more infant mortality and associated mental and physical attrition in women.

WOMEN IN HIGH-RISK PROFESSIONS

Women, as we know, are the traditional health providers in the home and also feature prominently in the alternative health professions as birth attendants and spiritual mediums. Moreover, in the modern health-care delivery system, women are over-represented in the treatment and care of people with AIDS as well as in the professions of midwifery and nursing.

The point therefore must be made that AIDS has not only increased women's burdens in the care of the terminally ill, but also risk of infection. For example, due to a number of well-known constraints, the majority of pregnant women either do not attend prenatal clinics and/or do not deliver in maternity wards. And even if they do, the absence of mandatory blood screening for pregnant women rules out a greater chance of AIDS detection. The result is therefore that midwives and birth attendants are clearly exposed to risks of AIDS infection.

An illustrative case was seen in a rural privately-owned maternity hospital in the research area where a pregnant woman came for prenatal care with an attendance card on which was clearly marked "HIV positive" by a Kampala-based hospital. The midwife on duty treated the woman and instructed her to transfer to a government hospital at the time of delivery. The midwife however explained that many such women came as emergency cases in labor without any card or without being known or diagnosed as having AIDS. It was also learned that although the government had distributed gloves, they were insufficient in quantity and in size, and that older midwives who had never used them in their lives were unwilling now to use them. They were therefore fatalistic about the risks of AIDS, although they continued to discharge or recommend transfer of any persons with AIDS to government or missionary hospitals.

As it is the practice in the government hospitals not to disclose people who are HIV positive and also to discharge the majority of these people, the burden of nursing people with AIDS, sometimes for a period of six months or more, is falling on women. Treatment risks are high, especially with traditional remedies that involve scarifications. Many women also reported that treating AIDS was trying, as it entailed considerable drainage of scarce human and material resources, and was not suited to traditional home management facilities. No wonder that some people with AIDS were known to have been abandoned alone in their homes.

Prostitution and bar-maid service are two professions at high risk for AIDS. More than anything, it is an indication of the height of economic despair that women in these occupations continue to operate even in AIDS-prevalent areas like Kalisizo and Kyotera. In Uganda as much as 86% of 186 barmaids screened in North Rakai district were found HIV positive in 1986.

THE CONDOM

Apart from abstinence from high-risk sexual behaviors, the proper use of condoms is considered to be the best protection against infection from AIDS. But perhaps because this is one method that shifts the burden of sexual and reproductive responsibility from the woman to the man, it has in the past never been aggressively promoted and marketed. Furthermore, men in Uganda have traditionally regarded condoms as detracting from their full sexual pleasure. In addition some women object to condom use by their partners out of fear that the condom can escape to the uterus and impair fertility or cause birth of deformed babies. However, there is evidence that among a small minority of young unmarried educated adults, a larger proportion of the men utilize condoms as a contraceptive measure against premarital pregnancy (Kisekka, 1976; Nichols, Ladipo, Paxman & Otolorin, 1986).

With the growing scare of AIDS, condoms promise to gain a high degree of acceptance. In Uganda, for example, where large free quantities of condoms were shipped, people even in the villages were quite well-informed about their use. Interestingly, women who were fearful of their husbands' resistance to "zero grazing" (monogamy in marriage) were in the habit of placing condoms in their husbands' pockets or overnight bags just as a necessary precaution against AIDS infection.

Corruption and the profit motive are so widespread, unfortunately, that condoms designated for free distribution to the public were nevertheless found in village shops, selling at a cost of five shillings each. Many other such free shipments disappeared from Uganda and were traded in the Bukoba district of Tanzania. Yet other packets of condoms which were deposited for free distribution at such places as private clinics or maternity hospitals were lying dormant as proprietors did not want to jeopardize their businesses by being associated with fertility control measures.

In spite of these constraints, one could conclude that in Uganda in centers of commercial sexual activities such as hotels and bars, there was evidence of growing condom use. This conclusion is based on widely reported findings of discarded used condoms around these premises, which children were habitually scavenging for and using as toy balloons. At the same time it appeared that there was a noticeable degree of misuse, as often people would borrow used condoms while some would wash and re-use them.

CONCLUSION

On the basis of a pilot assessment of the AIDS situation in Uganda, this paper has demonstrated the existence of AIDS as a major reproductive and sexual issue for women. It has argued that because of the traditional gender hierarchy and power relations in African societies, women are disproportionately· exposed to consequences of high-risk sexual behaviors by men, and at the same time have limited access to treatment resources and facilities. Additionally, by virtue of their reproductive, health providing, and management roles, women are not only exposed to the risks of AIDS but also bear the major concomitant psychosocial crises.

Policy

These findings point to a number of policy implications, some of which have been stated repeatedly, but with little or no effort at implementation.

First, there is need to popularize the condom to the general public and particularly to groups at high risk for AIDS. This cannot be overemphasized given the rising frequency of AIDS and other STDs. Although it is a male contraceptive, women contacts of men who engage in high-risk sexual behaviors have a vested interest in the use of condoms and need therefore to be enlightened to insist on its utilization as a prophylactic against AIDS, if not as a contraceptive.

Given the extent and magnitude of AIDS and its catastrophic sequelae, particularly to women, it is sound foresight for governments to subsidize the cost of condoms and to freely distribute them especially to the needy but economically deprived members of the population.

The AIDS situation necessitates a profound and radical approach from the current social management practices. In Uganda, as is imaginably the same in other hard-hit African countries like Rwanda, Zaire, etc., the care and management of people with AIDS should no longer be totally abandoned to their family and relatives. For it is clear that the amount and quality of care needed for people with AIDS are tremendous and they exact not only material but social and psychological tolls on the home health providers, an overwhelming majority of whom are women. There is therefore a need for the establishment of some new institutions, perhaps in the form of half-way hospitals where relatives can participate in the health care and management of their terminally-ill relatives along with hospital personnel.

It seems also justifiable and indeed a reproductive right that pregnant women who are under risk of AIDS should be screened and, if found positive, they should be counseled and given the option of a legal abortion.

Research

Among the relevant envisaged investigations is the focus on the relationship between sexual values and behaviors and spread and prevention of AIDS (Kisekka, 1988). These sexual variables run the gamut from taboos, etiquette, hygiene, and standards to types of sexual relationships and acts. Secondly, the community's classifications and perceptions of etiology and cure of AIDS are pertinent. Thirdly, the extent to which "tourist sex," the sexual adventures of tourists with partners abroad and its variant forms of sexual practices, have infiltrated the urban and youth categories, constitute an intriguing question for research.

Studies of prevalence rates are important and to be truly valid and meaningful they require a multidisciplinary approach involving the collaboration of social scientists with health professionals in executing clinic-based or epidemiological investigations in the communities. Related to this is the need to ascertain the extent and nature of self diagnostic medication, and self-referral.

Research should not only focus on people who have AIDS but on their significant others as well. The adaptation mechanisms in coping with this tragedy are relevant to the social rehabilitation and management of people with AIDS and their relatives and friends. The effect of the AIDS epidemic on dating, sexual, health seeking, and health delivery behaviors, as well as on marriage and family relations, pose crucial issues in family and medical sociology.

Research devoted to the acceptability of condom use is now more critical than at any other period in the history of reproductive health. Aspects of this research have been carefully delineated (Mundingo, 1987). They include determining the goals and norms of existing public health/family planning providers in order to assess whether the condom is acceptable to them since in their policy-making role they can facilitate or impede accessibility. Second, the service aspects of the condom need to be investigated in the sense that the attitudes of and problems encountered by service providers represent a major dimension of acceptability. For if these service providers do not distribute, recommend, sell or dispense the condoms, they remain unutilized. Lastly but most importantly is research focusing on users'/clients' perceptions of and experiences with the condom. This user perspective includes potential acceptability by non-users who intend to use the method; decision-related acceptability, that is, those who are currently faced with a decision; and experiential acceptability, involving people who have been using condoms for a defined period of time.

The details outlined by the WHO Task Force on Behavioural and Social Determinants of Fertility Regulation with particular reference to research on condom acceptability are concordant with our research interests. They suggest that research themes could be investigated within an operations research, focus group or special survey model and could be collaborative, comparative, prospective or retrospective. For researchers keen on operations research, a number of interventions are advanced:

   a. implementing special educational activities in a community;
   b. mobilizing — through special motivation — the support of community leaders and other influential people;
   c. utilizing commercial channels for the distribution of condoms (market vendors, small shops, etc.);
   d. retraining service providers to give more attention to condoms;
   e. testing ways to bring men into clinics (special hours, male staff to give advice on condoms, etc.). (WHO, 1987, p.3)

Finally, a reminder and point of emphasis concerns the fact that all our research endeavors in the Association of African Women for Research and Development (AAWORD) are guided by the motive and goal of redressing existing unfair gender hierarchies. The problem of STDs, as discussed in this paper, is a gender issue and is one replete with challenging research themes of theoretical and applied significance, which in a large measure represent our vision of a solution for this multifaceted and globally linked crisis.

REFERENCES

Brandenburg J.B. (1982). Sexual harassment in the university: Guidelines for establishing a grievance procedure. *Signs*, *8*, 320-336.
Crawford, R.J. (1980). Healthism and the medicalization of everyday life. *International Journal of Health Services*, *10*.

Hooper, E. (1987). Uganda fights "Slim Disease" with education. *People, 14,* 22.

Kisekka, M.N. (1976). Sexual attitudes and behaviour among students in Uganda. *Journal of Sex Research, 12,* 104-116.

Kisekka, M.N. (April, 1988). Socio-cultural beliefs and practices related to condom acceptability: A cross-national study among Hausa in Nigeria and Baganda in Uganda. Project proposal submitted to WHO Task Force on Behavioral and Social Determinants of Fertility Regulation.

Mundigo, A.I. (October, 1987). Acceptability of fertility regulation methods: Concepts and research needs. A discussion paper for Research Workshop on Condom Acceptability, Arush, Tanzania.

Mulinde-Musoke, S. (October, 1987). Slim is forcing people to change social habits. *The New Vision,* 10.

Nichols, D., Ladipo, O. A., Paxman, J.M., & Otolorin, E. O. (1986). Sexual behavior, contraceptive practice, and reproductive health among Nigerian adolescents. *Studies in Family Planning, 17,* 100-106.

Republic of Uganda Ministry of Health (Sep. 1988). AIDS Control Programme, *Monthly AIDS Surveillance Report.*

The Weekly Review (February 1989). Kenya, The Tenth Annual Medical Scientific Meeting.

WHO Special Programme of Research in Human Reproduction: Task Force on Behavioral and Social Determinants of Fertility Regulation (October, 1987). Paper circulated at Research Workshop on Condom Acceptability, Arusha, Tanzania.

Family Planning and Maternal Health Care in Egypt

Mawaheb T. El-Mouelhy

The process of development in any country depends basically on policy, people and resources. If the policy is sound, if most people are productive and if available resources are being used optimally, then a country is likely to develop and prosper. If, on the other hand, the policy is wrong, most people unproductive, and available resources are not being used properly with little effort to create additional or alternative resources, then the process of development in a country is not likely to move forward.

The human element is very important in this connection. The "people" factor plays a dramatic role and people naturally consist of both men and women. For people to be productive, they have to be basically healthy, and health — as defined by the World Health Organization — is a state of complete physical, mental and social well-being and not merely the absence of disease or infirmity.

In Egypt, more attention is now being given to the health status of women. Reproductive behavior of Egyptian women directly affects their health and well-being. Studies in Egypt have recently shown that pregnancy, labor and abortion kill 20-23% of all women

Mawaheb T. El-Mouelhy, MB, BCh (Ain Shams, Egypt), DRCPI (Dublin, Ireland), Medical Doctor — Egyptian, has ten years experience in Obstetrics and Gynaecology in Egypt, England, Saudi Arabia and Abu Dhabi. For the last three years she has been working as a physician with the Cairo Family Planning Association (CFPA) and is Director of the F.P. Model Center in Zeinhom, Cairo. She is involved in research on Women, Reproductive Health and Development in Egypt and is a member of the Arab Women Solidarity Association (AWSA), a feminist organization based in Cairo.

Requests for reprints may be sent to Dr. Mawaheb El-Mouelhy, Arab Women Solidarity Association, 4A, Dareeh Saad St., Off Kasr El-Eini St., Cairo, Egypt.

55

who die in their reproductive age (15-49) and produce many more disabilities some of which could be major and/or permanent (El-Mouelhy, 1987).

Family Planning consequently is a crucial preventive health measure for women in Egypt and it acts essentially by reducing the number of pregnancies for each woman, consequently reducing complications from pregnancy, labor and abortion. Pre-natal care is also very important for increasing the safety of the pregnancies by detecting high risk cases in time and dealing with them properly. It is clear that both family planning and pre-natal care are essential elements in preventing and reducing the number of deaths and disabilities among women in their reproductive years.

Egypt's population now is just over 50 million and increasing by almost 2.8% every year. The total fertility rate (the average number of live children born to a woman during her life time) is around 5 (Zurayk, 1988). The illiteracy rate for women in Egypt is more than 60% and their participation in the labor force is less than 6% (Zurayk, 1988). Women's low health status, which is already affected by repeated pregnancies and their complications, is complicated even further by some diseases prevalent among women such as anaemia and malnutrition. The social conditions make the picture look even worse by adding the amount of the daily work load the woman has to deal with. The large number of children the Egyptian woman has to care for, the hard daily work at home and the demands of the husband and family consume most of her time, leaving her with almost no time to care for herself and exposing her to both physical and mental stress. Given all these factors, how can a woman in Egypt be expected to share or be involved in the development of her community and country and raise sound and healthy children?

In 1980, a fertility survey in Egypt revealed that 53% of a sample of married women between the ages 15-49 did not want any more children and yet less than half of them were actually using contraceptives at the time of the survey. Why these women did not seek family planning despite their wish not to have more children is not a simple answer. More complicated factors—other than the simple wish—are involved and have to be fully understood to help increase family planning programs in the country. Social, cultural, economic and institutional factors are all important in influencing such programs.

A successful and powerful family planning program depends not only on the availability and the quality of the services provided to the women but also on the socioeconomic and cultural factors within the society as well as the extent of the official support given by the state to encourage these programs.

Socioeconomic and cultural factors can influence people's motivation to have smaller families. Family planning in turn, by helping to slow population growth, can ultimately improve people's socioeconomic standard.

The status of the woman in the areas of education, health, poverty, employment, the family, public life, and the community can be a crucial determinant in her being accepting of family planning. We need to understand the relationship between the status of women in society and their reproductive behavior as well as existing socioeconomic and cultural factors before attempting to improve or modify family planning programs.

Most of the women who come to our family planning clinic are poor, illiterate homemakers. Many of them moved from rural areas to Greater Cairo to join their husbands who are mostly non- or semi-skilled workers who could not find jobs in their places of origin and moved to the city in the hope of finding a job and a better life. Generally, our clients are women of low socioeconomic class. Some of their stories follow.

Fatima told me her story when she came to seek family planning advice. She is twenty now, married when she was fourteen and now has three children in three consecutive pregnancies, all delivered by Caesarean sections. She feels her health is deteriorating while the demands of her children, her husband and the in-laws who live with her are increasing and becoming a burden. She wanted to delay pregnancy after the second child but her husband and mother-in-law forbade her to use any contraception. "They want more children but I cannot go on," she said. "If they know I came here, my husband will divorce me. I have no school education and no support. What am I going to do with three little kids on my own?" We attempted to talk to the husband but he refused to talk to us, saying this was a personal matter. A few months later, Fatima came back, crying for help. Her husband had divorced her when she refused to have a fourth child. She was awarded custody of the children but received very little financial support and she is now desperate for a job and a place to live.

On the contrary, Laila, who is now thirty-eight and has eight children, was brought up to believe that the more children the woman has, the more attached and faithful the husband will be and the more secure the woman will feel. Her husband is working abroad and comes home only two months every year. Every time he comes home she gets pregnant, despite his wish not to have any more children. Laila and I had a long talk together, since her husband was trying to find a way to send his wife for an abortion—which is severely restricted in Egypt. He did not want additional children but Laila was adamant to have the child, and she came to me for pre-natal care. At her last visit, she told me that her husband divorced her a few weeks ago and got married to another woman where he works.

Ahlam, who is now forty with six children, has just had an intra-uterine device (IUD) inserted in our clinic. Today, with an anxious look on her face, she is asking me to take it out. Why? "My husband had been to the Friday prayer yesterday," she said, "The preacher addressed the people saying that family planning is forbidden by religion! My husband is a religious man; he asked me to have the IUD out today or he will throw me out on the street! I tried to discuss it with him but he told me the preacher knows better than anyone else."

Zeinab, who is now thirty-nine and has nine children, is happy, and so is her husband, who is a farmer. She is now pregnant for the tenth time! The couple is proud, saying that the pregnancy is God-given. Children for them are an asset. "One more child means two more helping hands," they say. "When they are eight or nine years old, we send them to work in the field, and they bring more money home."

Sabra, Zeinab's younger sister, who is thirty-three, has six children and the seventh is on the way. She has a similar view. "Why should we bother about the children's education, care, food and health?" she says, "It is the government's responsibility to care for them, don't they provide subsidized food, education and health care for every child no matter how many children we have? Why should we bother about the number of children we may have?"

Nawal is forty-one and has just had her fifth baby. A few months ago she went to a nearby family planning clinic to consult with the doctor on which contraceptive method to use. The doctor was not there and the nurse advised her to take the pill. Nawal was not examined; she was not even instructed how to use the pill. "I used it on and off when necessary," she said. "I thought that was the right way to use it, but I think I am pregnant." Nawal was ten weeks pregnant that day.

Mona is a teacher who comes from a small village just outside Cairo. She told me about the local Traditional Birth Attendant (TBA) in her village. Mona says the TBA discourages and disapproves of all methods of birth control, and warns the women in the village against it. Mona said the TBA is busy—with the high fertility rate in this village, she is becoming a rich woman!

Nadia, who is now twenty-nine and mildly diabetic, was married at age 13 and has five children. She could not go on the pill because of her medical condition and she tried other methods without success. She and her husband do not want any more children and she wants to be sterilized. She was referred to the hospital, but returned to the clinic a week later desperate and disappointed. She had been to four hospitals, all of which rejected her demand for sterilization. The reasons given by the doctors ranged from non-availability of the service to prohibition of the procedure for religious reasons.

The stories of the eight women described above reflect some of the weaknesses of our family planning and women's health programs. Illiterate, helpless, unsupported, powerless, neglected and insecure women will be able to rear healthy and sound children, but will not easily accept family planning or properly utilize the existing health services. The resulting over-population will impede Egypt's development and will delay improving the socioeconomic conditions of Egyptian women. A lot of work needs to be done to improve the status of women in Egypt. First, if family planning programs are to succeed in Egypt, equal opportunities in education and employment must be provided for girls and women, in order for women to increase their income, to fight against poverty, and to reduce their burden to give them more time for themselves. Amending the unjustified and backward laws connected with marriage, divorce and custody is crucial, and enforcing laws to stop child marriage, especially in rural areas, is of utmost importance.

On the other hand, it is essential to provide good quality maternal care and family planning services nationwide, taking into consideration the wider choice of different methods of contraception and easy accessibility to these services by women of all socioeconomic levels. Personnel who are trained to work in this field and who can handle both medical and social problems are vital.

The state can greatly contribute in promoting women's health programs by taking a more active role and improving the present policy. More entertaining and scientific messages against harmful traditional beliefs and practices through the media are needed to reach both women and men in the community. The state could also help by creating a system of incentives and disincentives through the traditional healers, community leaders, and religious institutions in order to establish people's motivation to have smaller families and to better improve their health.

REFERENCES

El-Mouelhy, M. (1987). Maternal mortality in Egypt. Cairo Family Planning Association.

Zurayk, H. (1988). Role of women in the socioeconomic development in Arab countries. *The Arab Future Magazine, 109*(3). Center for Arab Unity Research.

Perceptions on Communication
and Sexuality in Marriage in Zimbabwe

Marvellous M. Mhloyi

The definition of marriage in Zimbabwe, like in other African countries, lacks precision due to its protracted nature. The marriage process begins at that stage when the next-of-kin of the prospective bridegroom propose their son's marriage to the prospective bride. At that point, lobola, which comprises cash, heads of goats and cattle, is discussed. Payment of lobola takes a long period; sometimes the lobola of a woman's daughter can be used to pay up her mother's. Families differ on the criteria they use to declare the prospective spouses husband and wife. Liberal families accept the proposition by family members as an adequate step to declare their daughter married; conservative families may demand full payment. In some parts of the country it is culturally sanctioned not to pay lobola at once for to do so spells unhappiness possibly terminating in divorce. The point is, unlike the Western marriage which is pronounced at the wedding which occurs on a particular date, the African marriage is a process whose duration of completion ranges from a few months to years.

Marriage can be loosely defined as an arrangement that establishes a more or less enduring legally and/or socially sanctioned relationship between a man and a woman, and within which procreation — a young man's familial obligation to extend the lineage —

Dr. Marvellous M. Mhloyi is Chairman and Demography Lecturer in the Sociology Department, University of Zimbabwe. Her research interest and work is in fertility and family.

Requests for reprints may be sent to Dr. Marvellous Mhloyi, Chair, Department of Sociology, University of Zimbabwe, PO Box MP 167, Mount Pleasant, Harare, Zimbabwe.

61

takes place. Marriage occupies a central role in the security and prosperity of the lineage and is thus controlled by a generation of elders in the extended family system (McDonald, 1985; Mhloyi, 1987).

Since marriage is exogamous to the lineage, the payment of lobola (bridewealth) in exchange for women subordinates a woman who is perceived as an outsider to the kin group. A birth is thus a connecting link between the outsider and the lineage. In this marriage contract female fidelity is highly essential since infidelity increases the chances of having children who do not belong to the lineage, a situation warranting divorce. Since male infidelity is received as only consistent with men's most important function of extending the familial line, it enhances high fertility. Female sexual desire is abhorred while that for males is the sin-qua-non of manhood. This is also consistent with the expectation of female and not male virginity upon entry into the marriage contract. An obvious double standard characterized by male infidelity equated to the enhancement of the family and female infidelity equated to the destruction of the family is apparent.

This traditional form of maintaining a pristine lineage is gradually changing. Such changes can be more easily understood if viewed against a background of the basic evolution of societies specified by Weber and posited by McDonald (1985) as comprising three basic stages. The three stages can be described as traditional, transitional and modern. At the beginning of this continuum, the lineage is the principal unit of production and consumption. Hence it controls its members because it provides for their economic, physical and spiritual security.

At the middle of the continuum is a second form of social organization characterized by the preeminence of power at a higher level than that of lineage, ranging from tribe or lordship through industrialized nation states. At the other end of the continuum is the advanced capitalist mode of production characterized by urbanization, industrialization and individualism.

The meaning and basis of marriage change along this economic continuum. At the beginning of the continuum marriage has a passionate basis paced by economic considerations; hence it anchors in the extended family system. Since land is the economic base and belongs to the lineage, it is that lineage which has decision making power on matters of importance. A woman, an outsider, is powerless and can only enhance her survival within the family by her fidelity, fertility, and complete loyalty to the kin group. During the second stage characterized by modernization, education is often biased toward sons. This empowers the young male generation while the woman remains subordinate economically. However, with increased modernization at the third stage, including female education and women's consequent marketability in the modern labor market, the economic dependence for females is transformed into both financial and reproductive contributions. Women's sense of individualism increases, thus facilitating a more rational assessment of traditional mores including those which suppress their sexuality.

The transition from a traditional to a modern society is not paralleled by a shift from the double standard regarding spousal fidelity to a situation whereby extramarital sex is prescribed for both men and women. Modern society, however, is characterized by drastic changes in women's views about their own sexuality with a consequent increase in extramarital sex by women.

As women gradually loosen the social chains that tie them, men (their captors) attempt to maintain their grip by imposing severe punitive measures on "unfaithful" wives. Such measures include reprimands, severe battering, and even death.

The scenarios depicted above must not be erroneously perceived as comprised of personal antagonism between women and men, but rather as coordinated social systems deeply entrenched in the respective cultures — systems which cannot be mechanically and expeditiously changed. Granted, women are also members of this social system; thus they are also captors of themselves.

Zimbabwe is characterized by different degrees of these aforedescribed three stages. Urban areas are more characteristic of the transition from the second to the last stage. In the rural and most traditional society, there is a network of aunts and/or brothers-in-law through which problems relating to sexuality are communicated and solutions sought. However, it must be noted that this is indirect communication between spouses. The transitional stage is accompanied by increased family nucleation and disappearance of the communication channels typical of traditional societies. Such modernization fosters a more rational approach to life including sexuality—a development demanding direct communication between spouses. Lack of such communication may result in frustration and a consequent seeking of solutions outside the family; such a development can destabilize families.

This study focuses on the urban areas which represent the most developed (modernized) part of Zimbabwe. Thus, the attitudes towards extra-marital sex, of both women and men who were residents of Harare, the capital city of Zimbabwe, were solicited. Thirty males and thirty females were interviewed. An in-depth, open-ended questionnaire was administered to individuals, and to two focus group sessions—one female and the other male. Percentages were calculated from the sample of sixty respondents.

ACCEPTABILITY OF EXTRA-MARITAL SEX

Women and men were asked directly whether or not extra-marital sex was acceptable. Generally, extra-marital sex is more acceptable for men than for women. Approximately 42 percent and 27 percent of the men and women, respectively, view extra-marital sex as acceptable for men. Eight percent of male respondents accepted extra-marital sex among women while no woman did.

Conditions under which extra-marital sex by women is acceptable were solicited from women and men, respectively. According to women, the most justifiable reason for female extra-marital sex (having an affair) is male erectile difficulty. It should be noted that this reasoning is culturally derived. Traditionally male erectile difficulty and the consequent couples' infertility was solved by privately arranging extra-marital sex between women and their husband's next-of-kin.

The second condition under which extra-marital sex was perceived as acceptable was women's unsatisfied sexual needs. The most important reason was that men engage in extra-marital sex for long durations. Most women, approximately 80 percent, argued that men take female sexuality for granted. Women argued that men do not care about exciting their wives sexually. Consider this comment:

Ah; males are unfair, some just jump on you like a cork. Where are those foreplays typical of the good old days?

Another reason given for husbands' inability to satisfy their wives is drunkenness which all respondents associated with reduced sexual libido in men. Women also remarked that men cease to treat their wives as "ladies" once they are married. One woman, a homemaker, bitterly remarked:

My husband never tries to evoke that woman in me. No matter how dressed I am, I look the same to him. You only get surprised when another man comments that: 'if your husband were to drop you I could catch you before you hit the ground.'

Another homemaker added:

My husband consistently made me feel like I was no longer a woman with feelings. I had to have extra-marital sex to test whether or not I was still normal. To my surprise my partner expressed unmistaken enjoyment.

A number of women, including the focus group, argued that with modernization women are exposed to a number of options. They emphasize the fact that married women also want to be loved and entertained (women assume that their respective husbands do all this to their extra-marital sexual partners). Some women said that they met their husbands in public places but after marriage their husbands do not allow them to drink alcohol, and thus do not ever take them to such public places. Such women may resort to drinking alcohol with other male friends. They further argued that the most important reason for female extra-marital sex is not pecuniary but emotional. They contended that women are now capable of solving their own problems, and this is facilitated by their exposure to the wider community in urban areas and at work places.

It was generally argued that men are often defensive when they are not satisfying their wives sexually. One woman (a school teacher) remarked:

You know after two months of no sex I tried to arouse my husband sexually and he hastened to tell me that I had a disease of high libido which my parents had to treat. I was hurt and decided to treat myself.

Another reason given for extra-marital sex by women was the need for financial help. Some women are reported to "exchange sex for jobs." This is consistent with the argument that women, in traditional societies, are economically dependent on men, a dependence which may determine marital choices. With modernization, women become involved in the modern labor market which is dominated by their more educated, skilled and experienced male counterparts. Within that context, some women find themselves sexually vulnerable to men in exchange for jobs and/or promotions.

It should be clear from the foregoing discussion that there is some element of scapegoating by women who engage in extra-marital sex, i.e., men are always to blame. It is quite clear, and some women acknowledged this, that women have a sexuality which has to be satisfied. If that satisfaction (enjoyment) is not realized within marriage, some women will seek such satisfaction elsewhere. While the initial act might be a reaction to frustration, following the women's general argument, to the extent that such reaction minimizes frustration, such behaviour may become routine. The explanation for such a routine will be consistent, to a large extent, with the reasons men give for female extra-marital sex—the most obvious one being enjoyment accrued from behaving deviously and secretively.

It is interesting to note that men generally agreed to the validity of the reasons for female extra-marital sex given by women. They however added that some women will basically always be involved in extra-marital affairs. However, men also demonstrated a relatively high degree of naiveté regarding female sexuality. Consider these remarks:

A wife does not necessarily have to enjoy sex. Her function is to bear children. (clerk)

or

> Women are rarely unsatisfied by their marital sex; they engage in extra-marital sex mainly for pecuniary reasons. (university teaching assistant)

Reasons for the unacceptability of extra-marital sex by women are cultural. Both women and men reported that married women are not expected to engage in extra-marital sex so as to avoid "contaminating the lineage with foreign blood." A married woman is expected to be stable. This enhances not only her dignity but also her husband's. As hypothesized earlier, some respondents accepted male infidelity as consistent with polygamy, a behavior which, according to traditional beliefs, enhances fertility. (Note that while polygamy enhances a family's fertility it depresses females' individual fertility.)

There are more varied explanations for men's engagement in extra-marital sex. However, it is interesting to note that most of the reasons are related to men's sexuality. Most men, seventy percent, reported that men want a variety of sexual partners because it is exciting. One general worker remarked:

> Men are adventurous.

A university lecturer added:

> Men are always on an exploratory mission.

It was argued that some men are always searching, expecting to find women who can best satisfy their sexuality; the highest degree of satisfaction is often regarded as very high and rather illusive. Some men argued that men are generally lustful. It was also maintained that extra-marital sex by men is viewed as proof of their virility—some form of an obligation on the one hand and a "hobby" on the other.

Like women, men used some scapegoating to justify extra-marital sex. However, most of the explanations reflect society's perceptions regarding the woman's role in marriage. Some men reported that they engage in extra-marital sex during the postpartum abstinence period and also when the woman is menstruating. It was also reported that some men are not treated well by their wives to the extent that such men seek refuge with other women. One respondent elaborated on how his girlfriend helps him undress. Note that such behavior is mostly consistent with casual relationships which can be enhanced by such minor niceties. Extra-marital sex partners often attempt to outplay their boyfriends' wives so that they can be appreciated more and/or hopefully be married.

Like women, men also argued that male infidelity is necessitated by lack of marital sexual satisfaction. The reasons for the lack of satisfaction were that some women do not possess, nor try to acquire, those qualities which make women sexually attractive. Such qualities included long inner labia, brightly colored beads around the waistline, herbs to contract and "heat" the vagina, etc.

It was also reported that some women refuse sex with their husbands as a punishment; this forces men to engage in extra-marital sex. Temporary separations due to employment in urban areas while women reside in rural areas was also mentioned as an explanation for male infidelity. Surprisingly, women are expected to remain faithful in the rural areas under similar conditions, yet another indication of the assumption of female lack of sexual desire.

The overriding reason for male engagement in extra-marital sex given by women was the social sanction. Consider this remark:

Men are bulls. (homemaker)

Women also acknowledged the "adventure" in men; however, women typically did not understand the reason for such behavior. In particular, married women did not think that their husbands ignore them because they are not sexually exciting. It is interesting to note that prostitutes are quite aware of the reasons why they are more sexually attractive than the average married woman. The qualities which they give (from casual discussions with six prostitutes) coincide with some of the reasons, particularly those relating to sexual excitement, given by men for male engagement in extra-marital sex. For instance prostitutes maintained that they use herbs which contract and heat the vagina — an attribute which is supposed to be enjoyed by men (some men echoed this statement). They also reported that they wear beads, and that they are very active in bed.

"You have to make your man feel like a king; this is how we attract your husbands," a prostitute remarked.

KNOWLEDGE OF AND PRACTICE OF EXTRA-MARITAL SEX

A hundred percent of the male respondents reported that married women engage in extra-marital sex. However, only 20 percent of the women reported female engagement in extra-marital sex. There is almost unanimous agreement regarding male infidelity. Approximately 98 percent and 100 percent of men and women, respectively reported that men engage in extra-marital sex.

It is interesting to note, however, that 97 percent of the men (see Table 1) did not suspect their wives engaged in extra-marital sex. Three percent claimed not to know. This response is contradictory to the almost unanimous knowledge of married women's infidelity. Again this suggests the naiveté of men regarding their wives' situations and possible options. This may also be explained by men's refusal to face reality. Most husbands try to live with such reality by distancing from it. Thus, they reported that women in general engage in extra-marital affairs; their own wives do not. The closest to reality was a claim of lack of knowledge by 3 percent of the men.

The inconsistency of responses is also true for the actual engagement in extra-marital sex. Approximately 67 percent of the men compared with 3 percent of the women (see table) reported that they sometimes engaged in extra-marital sex. Four percent of the women reported that they have considered engaging in extra-marital sex.

Compare the normative values regarding extra-marital sex and actual behavior. While 58 percent of the men report that male infidelity is unacceptable, a higher percentage, 67 percent, report that they engage in extra-marital sex. This pattern is reversed for women; while 67 percent of the women reported that female infidelity is unacceptable, only 3 percent reported actual engagement in extra-marital sex and 4 percent considered it. It is clear that women are more puritanical in their sexual behavior than are men; this is consistent with societal expectations and with the aforementioned hypothesis that women are part of a social system that oppresses them.

TABLE 1. Results and Discussions. Summary of Results

	MALES			FEMALES		
	YES	NO	DEPENDS	YES	NO	DEPENDS
Female extra-marital sex acceptable	8.3	91.7	-	0.0	67.0	33
Male extra-marital sex acceptable	41.7	58.3	-	26.7	73.3	-
Married women have extra marital	0.0	100.0	-	20.0	80.0	-
Married men have extra marital	2.0	98.0	-	0.0	100.0	-
Suspects spouse etra marital sexual selection	-	96.5	-[1]	86.7	13.3	-
Sometimes engage in extra-marital sex	66.7	33.3	-	3.0	93.0	-[2]
Discuss with spouse your sexuality	66.7	33.3	-	33.3	66.7	-

[1] 3.5% of the men reported that they do not know whether or not their wives engage in extra-marital sex.

[2] 4% of the women reported that they have considered etra-marital sex.

PERCEIVED IMPACT OF EXTRA-MARITAL SEX
ON MARRIAGE

The respondents were asked about their possible reaction to their spouses' extra-marital sex. Most women, approximately 80 percent, reported that they would confront their husbands if they discovered that the men engaged in extra-marital sex. The remaining 15 percent reported that they would caution their husbands, while the rest were indifferent.

Men were more drastic in the measures they would take should they discover that their wives engaged in extra-marital sex. Approximately 60 percent stated that they would divorce their wives, 20 percent would severely beat their wives, while 18 percent would severely caution their wives, and 2 percent would simply express their disappointment and ask for a change in behavior. It is interesting to note that the reactions by men to their wives' extra-marital sex were similarly perceived by both women and men. Approximately 80 percent of the women maintained that extra-marital sex was the only justifiable reason for divorce. A significant number of women, 10 percent, spontaneously responded that their husbands would "lynch" them if they were known to engage in extra-marital sex. While it may not be necessarily true that the women would be killed, the consequences would be quite severe. The fact that female infidelity faces more drastic punitive measures may partly explain the lower proportion of women reporting actual engagement in extra-marital sex. Yet it also suggests that some women may engage in extra-marital sex in a more clandestine and secretive manner in comparison with men. Such practice may result in more intimate relationships which may inflict a greater negative impact on the marriage.

Respondents were asked about the possible impact of extra-marital sex by either spouse on the marriage. Regarding extra-marital sex by men, it was generally agreed that family resources, diverted to extra-marital partners, deprive the family of necessary support. It was believed that women who are involved in extra-marital affairs do not pay enough attention to their families; in particular they do not respect their husbands. It was generally agreed that extra-marital sex leads to marital disruption.

It was also generally agreed that men have always engaged in extra-marital sex; however, it was noted, as well, that extra-marital sex by women is on the increase. Asked what should be done about this situation the respondents suggested that spouses must learn to communicate about their sexuality to each other. Some respondents acknowledged the fact that such communication is not culturally normative and suggested that marriage counselling organizations should be established.

Granted the respondents' articulation of the need to communicate, how many respondents behave in the manner they suggest? Apparently the data tend to show that there is relatively minimal discussion of sexuality between spouses. Approximately 67 percent and 33 percent of the men and women, respectively, reported that they discuss their sexuality with their spouses. One would expect that approximately the same percentage of women and men would report discussion. The inconsistency shown by the data is difficult to interpret. A substantial proportion of women, 25 percent, reported that their husbands sometimes complain about how sexually unexciting they are. One may thus point out that men may consider such complaints to be "discussion." It was also added that women are not expected, culturally, to express sexual dissatisfaction which leaves the complaints as unidirectional, a situation which stifles communication and leads to frustration.

CONCLUSION

Harare is a modern city, infrastructurally. The transition from tradition to modernization, however, is not paralleled by the dissolution of a double standard regarding male and female sexuality. Yet the urban setting enhances family nucleation, thereby eroding the communications and support of the traditional extended family. It also facilitates the diffusion of ideas, including those inimical to marital stability. This urban setting also improves the status of women as they get involved in the labor market. With the increased exposure to new ideas and a wider community, women are beginning to question some of the traditional customs and mores regarding their sexuality and that of their male counterparts.

Against this background, it was generally observed that married couples engaged in extra-marital sex. The most important reason given for men's extra-marital sex was their socially sanctioned sense of "adventure." Women were reported to engage in extra-marital sex as a reaction to their husbands' attitudes towards them. The most fundamental explanation given for extra-marital sex was lack of marital sexual satisfaction. While women and men tended to scapegoat each other, it was clear that there is complacency about marital sexuality by both men and women. Married couples do not make an effort to understand and fulfill each others' sexuality; men are however worse than women in this respect.

It is also true that both women and men, once involved in extra-marital sex, enjoy it. Yet both tend to hide evidence of extra-marital sex from their own spouses. Both parties have complaints against the other, but complaints are minimally discussed while solutions are sought outside the marriage. Extra-marital sex by women is perceived to be on the increase and also more disruptive to the marital union than that of men; however, it must be understood that women are part of the social system whose functioning they contribute to. It is also incumbent upon women not to accept the traditional attitudes towards female sexuality. Women must attempt to assert their sexuality; however, such an assertion must be carefully articulated to avoid negative reactions from men and society at large.

It is important that women and men discuss sexual issues with their marital partners; such a development would minimize marital dissatisfaction and would be at least a first step toward the attainment of gender-equality.

REFERENCES

McDonald, M. (1985) *The Family System*. New York: Academic Press.
Mhloyi, M. (1987) "Couples perceptions about family formation-changes and prospects: The case of two rural settings in Zimbabwe" (Working Paper).

Bereavement and Stress in Career Women

Wilhelmina Kalu

SUMMARY. Several studies on the role of individuals and groups in social support networks indicate that such networks are instrumental in preventing depression and low morale as the result of major life events. In several African countries the existence of a strong kin-group relationship and communal style of living nurtures the proliferation of a social support network. This article explores the operation of significant individuals and groups for widowed women within the contemporary Nigerian context.

Stress theory views major life events (e.g., death in the family unit, divorce and child birth) as stressful and important in creating conditions for various somatic and psychological disorders (Greenblatt, 1978). This article will focus specifically on bereavement as a stressful life event. In the case of marital couples, bereavement deprives a spouse of a life-long partner, and the surviving spouse enters into a new role in life. Practices associated with mourning and bereavement in several societies and cultures mean that the process disproportionately affects women. In Africa, for instance, the prolonging of grief is culturally imposed on widows but not widowers (Amadiume, 1987). Bereavement therefore has stressful qualities in terms of the nature of grief, desolation over the loss of a loved one, and the inevitable acquisition of a new status in life as a widow or widower (Stroebe & Stroebe, 1983).

The buffering hypothesis states that a close interpersonal rela-

Dr. Kalu is Senior Lecturer in Educational Psychology and Special Education. She works as a child and family therapist and in child advocacy programs. Dr. Kalu serves in several national and international psychological associations. She has been in the academic field for fourteen years and is married with four children.

Requests for reprints may be sent to Dr. Wilhelmina J. Kalu, Dept. Education, University of Nigeria, Usuka, Nigeria.

75

tionship can serve to buffer individuals against the negative impact of stressful life events. This has been explored by Western clinical researchers and by those interested in social support network functions (Caplan, 1974; Cobb, 1976; Stroebe & Stroebe, 1983). The social support networks lessen the deleterious effect of stress and isolation (Lowenthal & Haven, 1968), and provide emotional support in terms of contributing to positive image, self-worth and reinforcement of desirable coping mechanism in the adjustment process (Burch, 1972). Support networks are also essential in the process of ventilation of anguished feelings such as are experienced in bereavement (Kirwen, 1979). They help to curtail prolonged or excessive grief and irrational despair (Clayton, Halikas & Maurice, 1971).

In most Western cultures social support network formations are being encouraged to help bereaved persons cope with the process of grief. Psychologists, counsellors and social workers may be involved to help identify possible friends, relatives, groups or acquaintances to help a bereaved married person during and after the burial of a spouse. In several situations, friends may be willing to help but are constrained by lack of time to spare for such a person (Briscoe & Smith, 1975; Caplan, 1976).

In several African societies such as Nigeria, however, the bereavement process is marked by several cultural landmarks as part of the celebration of transition into another life role (Kirwen, 1979). There is an abundant social support network including relatives on the mother's and father's sides of lineage, social clubs, church, town and community associations, and people of all ages. All individuals constituting the social support network are expected to participate in major life events affecting group members. Their number, function and participation in the event create several problems including lack of a centralized decision making process and lack of control over various activities of the groups. This may mean that stressful conditions are introduced into the experience of the bereaved. Cultural dynamics pertaining to widows, for example, weeks of confinement in a house before and after burial, and receiving treatment as if guilty of the death of one's husband, intensify these conditions beyond that experienced by bereaved men. What therefore occurs is a situation in which cultural practices collude with activities of social support networks to make life uncomfortable for the widow over a lengthy period.

SOME CHARACTERISTICS
OF CONTEMPORARY AFRICAN WIDOWS

Several studies indicate that the age at the time of bereavement has an impact on the severity of depressive symptoms (Maddison, 1969; Parkes, 1970). Young widows or those who are widowed before the age of 45 years experience difficulty in coping with grief in the first month of bereavement (Blanchard, Blanchard & Becker, 1976). A large percentage of African widows are young due to several factors, for example, early age of marriage for girls, marriage to older men, migration, and wars (Obbo, 1980). A recent study indicates that over 60% of widows are under 40 years of age (Okoro, 1988). (See Table 1.)

Since most African women are generally in employment in the labor force (Di Domenico, 1982), most widows (70%) are gainfully employed outside the home (Okoro, 1988). (See Table 2.) Thus youthful age and occupational roles appear as major factors in widowhood in contemporary African society. The young widow is often inexperienced in several aspects of life. She is faced with a

TABLE 1. Age of Widows in a 1987 Survey of Local Social Welfare Clients (N = 75)

Age Range	Frequency	%
20-30	30	40
30-40	20	26.7
40-50	15	20
50 and	10	13.3

TABLE 2. Career Occupation of Widows in a 1987 Survey of Local Social Welfare Clients

Occupation	Number of Widows	%
Full-time Homemaker	25	33.3
Farmers	20	26.7
Public Service Workers	5	6.7
Petty Traders	15	20
Child Minders	10	13.3

future of years of life ahead as a woman, but with the label of widow as common reference in social circles. She also has a life of economic independence and achievement to think about. She has to meet financial obligations to the self and the extended family. These are additional stressors involved in the immediate bereavement process and the future of adjustment to life as a widow.

STRESS WITHIN THE BEREAVEMENT
AND MOURNING PROCESS IN AFRICAN CONTEXT

Various practices and rites surround the celebration of death in African societies (Ekejiuba, 1984; Kirwen, 1979; Leith-Ross, 1965). Generally death is a celebration of transition into a higher status of life as an ancestor and therefore marked with drumming, singing, dancing, entertainment and ceremony. The focus of the discussion will, however, be on the widow and her stress in the mourning process within the contemporary urbanized setting.

Mourning often starts in Nigeria with a flurry of activities. There is a rush of people to the home of the bereaved person. The gathering of the crowd of friends, neighbors, and relatives begins within minutes or hours of the spouse's death. In Nigeria, the crowd of those seeking to show sympathy and to help turns quickly into throngs of sympathetic mourners. This continues day and night until the corpse is conveyed from the mortuary to the village of origin, the usual place of burial. A distinction is made between the place of residence for employment purpose and the "original home," the village of ancestry. The latter is the traditional place of burial, for an eternal rest among kin. Burial in towns and urban places is practiced on a small scale where economic hindrances prevent taking the body to the village home.

The friends and relatives comfort the widow in her grief and shock and ensure that she neither endangers her life with excessive grieving nor is over-burdened with other routine duties. The social support network therefore takes over the care of children, household chores, and errands connected with funeral announcements and arrangements. There is no particular order of assignment to groups, except that relatives are given precedence in the choice of roles and in making decisions. The widow, however, continues to grieve and cry often out of dread of demands made of the widowhood process. She has to cope with the demands of groups to which she or her husband belonged. These include social, religious and kinship groups.

In most traditional African societies, the extended or kin family (and not the nuclear family) owns the body of the dead person (Amadiume, 1987). The kin family of the bereaved husband exercises complete control over the corpse. It decides on the place and process of burial. Since the woman is a property of her husband's family according to Nigerian marriage rites, she is expected to submit to the dictates of his family. She may, however, have close sympathizers among them who support some of her rights. This is especially useful because the widow is asked to perform several traditional rituals of mourning at specified dates. These include the shaving off of her hair (Amadiume, 1987). This is a major area of disagreement between contemporary widows, who are career women, and the kin group.

The widow is expected to be available for consultation by the kin group at all hours, to receive all visitors who come to sympathize with her, and to cooperate fully with the husband's family. A few intimate friends therefore stay around her and make sure she gets rest whenever possible. These friends try to help her to compromise between traditional demands and the reality of contemporary changes. They keep her aware of her future responsibilities and the possibility of exploitation. They are also present for support and protection against excessive mourning when the corpse arrives at the village home.

Witch-hunting or scapegoating after a death is common in African societies (Amadiume, 1987). Witch-hunting refers to a process of searching for who is responsible for an unfortunate or tragic event such as death of a spouse. The African belief in evil spirits and forces directs attention to search for a person or agent through which an evil activity is made manifest. The person must be exposed and punished. The mourning period is the opportunity for any member of the husband's family who has been aggrieved at some point by the behavior of the widow in the past, to get even. Such persons are free to scold her, for instance, on the pretence that she did not treat the husband well when he was alive. The widow has to remain silent since she is expected to do little or no talking, let alone quarrel while her husband is not yet buried. The verbal insults are made directly or through proverbs, idioms and sarcasm. Clinical experiences indicate that these are very painful experiences for many widows. A group of intimate friends helps to soothe feelings through such periods. But there are also instances of physical abuse, like spitting on the woman or shaving her head bald against her will. There are reports of widows being made to eat out of broken plates, confined to wretched small rooms, or made to sit and sleep on bare floors for days (Amadiume, 1987). At a seminar in 1987 on Nigerian widows by the Media Women's Association of Nigeria, it was pointed out that most communities consider a woman guilty of her husband's death until proven innocent.

Stress from financial commitments are also common in the mourning process, although the kin family is expected to defray most of the financial costs involved. The constant flow of visitors into the house of the widow involves the hiring of chairs, tables for seating, electric wiring of premises and seating areas for improved illumination (especially for night vigils). There is need to provide traditional kola (a sign of welcome) and other refreshments for visitors, especially those who have come long distances. The many relatives who move into the home as helpers when it is used as a base for making the traditionally elaborate funeral arrangements have to be fed daily. There is little privacy, as every item in the home is put to public or communal use and damages are incurred in the process. There are also several other costs associated with fulfilling traditional rites and obligations by the widow.

The contemporary Nigerian widow is under stress not so much from the loss of the spouse but from the demands of a large and sometimes unwieldy group of significant others who participate in the funeral process. There is the dread of the late husband's relatives as the "powerful others" in the circumstance. It is a period of great unease with no clear guidance on meaningful behaviors. The objectives of several demands are often not clear and thus conflicting. The behavior of the groups involved in the process is not always complimentary or cooperative. Several situations within the mourning process are therefore unpredictable. Small consultation groups keep emerging and realigning themselves in the decision making processes.

UNEASY INDEPENDENCE
IN THE POST BURIAL PERIOD

There is generally a short period of confinement after the burial of a spouse in most African traditions. This confinement is usually done only once. It entails avoiding all public appearances (like going to the market, shops, church, or place of work; Amadiume, 1987). It is considered essential for rest after the rigors of the funeral process, as a sign of respect to the dead person, and as a period in which to make initial plans for the future of the widow and her children. It is also a period in which the widow receives several kin and official condolence groups.

The contemporary nature of dual residency, the village and urban homes, however, demands two periods of confinement. In both situations there are a series of visits from friends, groups, and colleagues. The confinements therefore imply obtaining a fairly lengthy period of absence from the place of work. The widow and her children are not allowed to spend a night elsewhere within the one-year period of mourning. This is a sign of respect to the dead spouse and also creates a period of isolation from regular extra-familial social interactions. This, however, combines with the tapering off of visitors over the months after burial to start a period of unanticipated serious isolation for the widow.

The widow therefore finds the return to social interaction with groups difficult at the end of the one-year mourning period. She is still considered part of her late husband's family, on account of the children of the marriage or until she gets remarried. Several clinical experiences indicate that part of the problem may come from the widow while a substantial proportion is from groups within the social support network.

In the absence of a well-articulated will to cope with the complex extended family system, there are often court processes as the result of the spouse dying intestate. This puts the widow and children on one side of the conflict and kin family on the other side with other groups choosing to identify with either side. It also affects the nature of regular income and therefore curtails financial commitments outside the home.

Some widows avoid appearing attractive in social gatherings for fear of being despised as searching for another husband too early. They therefore deliberately limit appearance in social gathering. Others find that celebrations and gatherings with intimate friends bring back painful reminiscences. These dampen their joy or increase their depression.

But for a number of widows there is an awakening to another kind of reality. Female friends feel uncomfortable inviting them to parties out of the fear of contamination by widowhood. There is uneasiness about the widow becoming dependent on a friend's husband for several of her problems in a male-dominated society. This may trigger suspicion of an extra-marital affair. Thus the post-burial and mourning period develop into a period of isolation and stress as the result of adjustment to a new status in life.

CASES OF BEREAVED CAREER WOMEN

A few cases selected from widowhood situations of friends and acquaintances residing in urban settings may help to illustrate the areas of stress within the bereavement process in contemporary contexts.

Case 1

Ngozi is a highly educated woman in her forties. She is articulate, fashion conscious and noted to be a quick-tempered person among her colleagues. She does her work well and is strict with subordinates. She is aware that she is not well-liked in her workplace but she has a satisfying family life and her goal is to excel in her career.

Ngozi places a lot of emphasis on what enhances her professional development. Thus she does not easily join traditional women's groups and associations in the town. She is also not a member of religious groups. She circulates among few intimate friends and professional groups and is involved in the activities of her three young children.

Her husband was a likeable person who got on well with subordinates and professional colleagues. At his death she was shattered but determined not to succumb to the loss and the traditional mourning processes. She has considered the experiences of contemporary widows as victims of deliberate acts of wickedness or communal assault. Thus she reacted quickly. She limited the flow of visitors to her home. She specified that they should not sing, talk loudly, or share laughter among themselves. Sympathizers were uncomfortable with several of her demands but she was convinced that compromises should come from others in order to allow her to handle the loss in her own way. Ngozi insisted on having her way over and above decisions of the kin throughout the funeral process.

Ngozi was a prime target for accusations from her husband's relatives. She held her peace when accused of ill-treating her spouse while he was sick. She gave several conditions concerning her welfare under which she would agree to a confinement period in the village. After the burial she allowed only individual or representatives of groups to call for condolence visits instead of the usual whole contingent of group members. In a matter of weeks her home was quiet and she was living in isolation, apart from interactions at the work place. She was rarely invited to functions which she avoided as a distraction from the care needed by her children who had lost their father. She was determined to maintain the same lifestyle that she and the children enjoyed prior to the death of her spouse. She was therefore caught in a host of activities each day that left her stressed. She experienced insomnia, prolonged grief and anger at both God and her late husband. She blamed friends for being too quick in abandoning her and lacking tolerance of her behavior under bereavement.

Case 2

Ama married in her teenage years. The marriage produced no children for several years. The husband was loving, supportive and unperturbed by the lack of children. Relatives, however, were unkind to Ama, seizing her property whenever possible in the village with the explanation that she had no offspring on which to use it. Ama was miserable until she became pregnant in her 30s, a few years before the death of her husband.

Both Ama and her husband belonged to several groups and associations, some jointly and others individually. They have been sensitive to social, religious, financial and host of kin group obligations. They were, for instance, involved in educating several relatives and helped some to acquire their own houses when the husband's consultancy firm prospered. At the death of the husband there was a long stream of visitors from the social support network. They were taken care of in the traditional way. Friends were generally helpful and supportive while relatives looked for several opportunities to get themselves shares of the late husband's acquisitions.

Despite the warmth shown her during the mourning period, Ama found herself isolated by close friends. She was sad at their suspicion when she received some individually for consultation, or visited those men she thought could help with special problems she encountered. Several relatives of her husband were not satisfied with their share of inheritance and made demands on her. Ama was under stress and uncertain from whom to seek advice. She faced a major handicap of having limited knowledge of her husband's agreement with partners of his firm. Hostility developed. At the same time she was holding a major responsibility in her workplace and her boss was unrelenting in the pressure on her to perform at work.

DISCUSSION OF THE CASES

The cases illustrate two of several different patterns of reaction to stress during widowhood. The psychological reactions within the adjustment process have not received serious research considerations in Africa. The nature of support groups and their operations have not been closely studied. These support groups are generally allowed to operate simultaneously and at their own volition leading to various reactions and counter reactions from each other and from the widow. This breeds an inevitable dread of widowhood and the mourning process. What is foremost in the mind of people is the need for legal provisions to alleviate undesirable consequences of socio-economic problems (human rights) associated with widowhood.

Many women consider widowhood problems as given, unsurmountable, and to be endured. Seeking counseling and therapeutic help is not a common practice and there is a fear of further antagonism of the kin group. In addition, widowhood problems are intricately embedded in the package of women-marriage-inheritance issues (considering cultural practices and modern reality). This means that the focus needs to be shifted to the long-range political solution associated with the legal rights of women.

In the midst of this confusion widows resort to different courses of action. A common feature is stress in the determination to handle or relate to groups in the social support network. In the case of Ngozi there was a rejection of the social support network despite its importance and usefulness. Her concern about the effect of her behavior on her children was valid.

Ngozi's refusal to cooperate with groups in her social support network, especially her kin family, was not an acceptable course of action to them. Ngozi's confusion is evident in her complaint about lack of laws to help her confront widowhood demands on her from the extended family. At the same time she was compelled to use the services of a lawyer in any situation she considered a threat.

On the other hand, Ama needed the services of a good law firm in addition to therapy. She needed such a firm to handle her affairs concerning her late husband's estate. Many of the requirements that are made from the courts will be considered as hostile action in the

African context by relatives. Ama therefore resorted to handling each situation on a personal basis. This was an awkward procedure and she approached the law rather belatedly. At the same time, friends gave her advice and she was subsequently overwhelmed by her problems. She had expected the worst in widowhood and was caught in a self-fulfilling prophecy.

Ama needed several sessions of counseling to provide relief from the stress she was experiencing. She also needed to continue to be assertive, to determine her priorities and to learn how to implement decisions thoroughly without yielding to pressure later on from family members. Ama had to learn how to terminate helping relationships after an objective had been achieved.

CONCLUSION

It is evident that the extended family and communal style of living have generated additional support groups. These have been added to the traditional kin groups whose usefulness has been appreciated over the years and who have more or less remained unquestionable in their right to operate. However, the merging of traditional and contemporary relationships between persons and groups can be problematic. The possibility of involvement in an unwieldy support group network has not been given serious consideration. There are therefore few guidelines on adaptive courses of action for women within such a relationship. In contemporary widowhood this issue is fundamental to recovery from mourning and the adjustment process. High social interaction appears to be more stressful in bereavement and it is likely that the widow may be giving more support to significant others than receiving reciprocal support in return.

REFERENCES

Amadiume, I. (1987). *Male daughters, female husbands: Gender and sex in an African society*. New Jersey: Zed Books Ltd.

Blanchard, C. G., Blanchard, E. B., & Becker, J. V. (1976). The young widow: Depressive symptomatology throughout the grief process. *Psychiatry, 39*, 394-399.

Briscoe, C. W., & Smith, J. R. (1975). Depression in bereavement and divorce:

Relationship to primary depressive illness: A study of 128 subjects. *Archives of General Psychiatry, 32,* 439-443.

Burch, J. (1972). Recent bereavement in relation to suicide. *Journal of Psychosomatic Research, 16,* 361-366.

Caplan, G. (1974). *Support systems and community mental health.* New York: Behavioral Publications.

Caplan, G. (1976). The family as a support system. In G. Caplan & A. Killelie (Eds.). *Support systems and mutual help* (pp. 19-36). New York: Grune and Stratton.

Clayton, P. J., Halikas, J. A., & Maurice, W. L. (1971). The bereavement of the widowed. *Diseases of the Nervous System, 32,* 597-604.

Cobb, S. (1976). Social support as a moderator of life stress. *Psychosomatic Medicine, 38,* 300-314.

Di Domenico, C. M. (1982). Role strain and working mothers in an urban centre in Nigeria: Some implications for mental health. In Erinosho, O. A. and N. W. Bell, (Eds.) *Mental health in Africa* (pp. 228-236). Ibadan, Nigeria: University Press.

Ekejiuba, F. (1984). Women in Igbo religious system. Paper presented at Institute of African Studies Congress, University of Nigeria, Nsukka.

Greenblatt, M. (1978). The grieving spouse. *American Journal of Psychiatry, 135,* 43-47.

Kirwen, M. C. (1979). African Widows. New York: Mary Knoll Orbis Books.

Leith-Ross, S. (1965). African Women (A study of the Ibo of Eastern Nigeria). London: Routledge and Kegan Paul.

Lowenthal, M. E., & Haven, C. (1968). Interaction and adaptation: Intimacy as a critical variable. *American Sociological Review, 33,* 20-30.

Maddison, D. (1969, January 9). The consequences of conjugal bereavement. *Nursing Times,* 50-52.

Obbo, Christine (1980). African women: Their struggle for economic independence. London: Hutchinson & Co. Ltd.

Okoro, N. N. (1988). The socio-economic adjustment of widows in a changing society and social services available: A case study of Arochukwu community. Unpublished Diploma Social Work Thesis, University of Nigeria, Nsukka.

Parkes, C. M. (1970). The first year of bereavement: A longitudinal study of the reaction of London widows to the death of their husbands. *Psychiatry, 33,* 444-467.

Stroebe, M. S., & Stroebe, W. (1983). Who suffers more? Sex differences in health risks of the widowed. *Psychological Bulletin, 93,* 279-301.

Nigerian Women's Quest
for Role Fulfillment

Judith D. C. Osuala

SUMMARY. This article examines the nexus between Nigerian women's struggle for role fulfillment and adult education. The women in the study experienced staggering disparities between their illiteracy and their optimal role expectations. As middle-aged workers and mothers of large families, they undertook self-initiated study in adult evening classes. Through the modality of the Focus Group Discussion Method (FGD), the women revealed their role-related problems and the specific ways by which adult education had empowered them to be self-actualizing in their traditional roles.

INTRODUCTION

Women everywhere experience tensions related to their need for role fulfillment. Women's demanding roles as wife, mother, worker and organization member tend to dissipate their energies and afford them little opportunity to realize their full potential. In countries like the United States, some women can learn to resolve their tensions and role conflicts through psychological therapy. This option is simply not available, however, to the vast majority of women in a developing country like Nigeria. Instead, these women

---

Judith D. C. Osuala, PhD, is Senior Lecturer in the Department of Adult Education, University of Nigeria in Nsukka, Nigeria. She is Coordinator of the Women's Network of Nigerian National Council for Adult Education and author of many publications including, "Extending Appropriate Technology to Rural African Women," "Basic Education Modules for Nigerian Women," and the literacy books, *Literacy and Numeracy Primer in English* and *Let's Be Healthy*.

Requests for reprints may be sent to Dr. Judith Osuala, Dept. Adult Education, University of Nigeria, Nsukka, Nigeria.

may turn to adult education as a means of enhancing their multiple roles.

This article focuses on adult education as an agent of role fulfill-ment for Nigerian women. It relates the findings of a base-line study carried out in 1988 with women who attended evening adult education classes in Nsukka, a medium-sized university town in Nigeria.

The primary objective of the adult education program is the prep-aration of adults for the First School Leaving Certificate. The pro-gram is intended for men and women who were unable to obtain a grade school education in childhood. The adults purchase their own textbooks and pay a monthly fee for attending the classes. The study concentrated on: (a) the characteristics of the women partici-pants; (b) their motivation for attending the classes, as it related to their role needs; and (c) their assessment of the benefits derived from the classes.

The Focus Group Discussion method (FGD), which is currently being used in socio-cultural and anthropological studies (Aubel, 1988; Muganzi, 1988), was used in the research. The FGD method elicits indepth information from a small (focus) group in the relaxed atmosphere of an informal discussion. The researcher directs prede-termined questions to the entire group and tape records the ensuing discussion. Objective data such as age at marriage, husbands' occu-pations, etc., are obtained through a show of hands.

The FGD method is as flexible as that used in unstructured inter-views in that the researcher's direct and indirect questions can be raised at appropriate times during the discussion. The group dyna-mism encourages participants to converse freely with their peers on the topic. The FGD method reveals the inner feelings, values and motives of people which could not be easily extracted from formal interviews or questionnaires. It is also appropriate for illiterate groups such as the women in the present study. The essence of the FGD method is the discovery and reporting of both common and divergent views and practices of the research sample.

Permission was obtained from the Local Government Authorities to meet with the women participants from 7:00 to 9:00 P.M. on weekday evenings when the classes were normally held. All of the 62 women in attendance in the five existing adult education centers were used as research subjects. They were placed by the researcher in groups of 10 to 13 and discussion questions were posed. The women were encouraged to contribute their ideas and they participated enthusiastically. The sessions were tape-recorded.

CHARACTERISTICS OF THE WOMEN

The purpose of this aspect of the research was to ascertain the demographics of the women who left their homes to attend adult classes every evening. Demographics gathered included marital status, age, parity, educational background, occupation and husband's occupation.

Through a show of hands it was discovered that all of the women participants were married with the exception of three who were young women still living with their parents. The ages of all of the women ranged from 18 to 46 with a mean age of 32.4 years. More than half of the women (65%) had from five to eight children, with the majority having six. The women had married between the ages of 12 and 20 with most marrying at 17. A large number of them had given birth to their first child the following year in order to confirm their fertility. Producing children is one of the women's major roles. It is a vital function because without male offspring, neither the women nor their husbands can claim essential cultural rights or privileges within this patrilineal society. Due to their early marriages and frequent child-bearing at a young age, it can be understood why, after 15 or 20 years of marriage, most of them had large families.

With regard to their entering educational level, 82% of the women said that they had not attended school previously. Many of them explained that they had come from large families and their fathers had trained only the sons. Their rationale for not training their daughters had been that "women's education only ends in the kitchen," or "the husband's family will enjoy the benefits." Others, who were the oldest daughters, had been kept at home to assist their overburdened mothers. The fathers had also married their daughters off while young to prevent them from being "spoiled" as this would have brought shame to the family.

Most of the women said that they had married men who held

semi-skilled jobs such as night watchman, laborer, messenger and mason, although a few husbands were teachers or lecturers. All of the women worked at low level jobs. Nearly half (48%) were market traders, while the next largest number (10%) were hair dressers. Others were seamstresses, farmers, church and hospital workers, and cooks. These were the only types of occupations available to them since they did not possess the primary school certificate.

The women who were market traders said they sold food items in the spacious outdoor market in the center of Nsukka town. They usually arrived at the market early in the morning to buy fresh food items "wholesale" and then sell them at a retail rate the remainder of the day. At other times they travelled to remote rural markets to purchase items for sale. In either case, their profit margin was seldom commensurate with the labor involved. A good number of the hairdressers and seamstresses said they also plied their trades inside the market.

MOTIVATION OF THE WOMEN
FOR ENROLLING IN ADULT EDUCATION

When the women were asked their reasons for joining the adult education classes, there was an explosion of eager responses at all of the centers. The high points of the ensuing discussions are categorized below as relating to the women's roles as: (a) members of social groups; (b) workers; (c) wives and mothers; and (d) self-actualizing persons.

Social Role

A majority of the women expressed their desire to be literate in order to take part fully in the social organizations to which they belonged. They voiced their chagrin at dressing in their best clothes to attend meetings and then being unable to sign their names or to join meaningfully in the proceedings. Some of them aspired to hold executive positions in order to write the minutes of the meetings, to call roll, or to count the contribution like the educated members.

One of the illiterate women related how she had accidentally been elected President of her town union. She was so discomfited by her inability to read her Secretary's minutes or to manage the affairs of the union that she had promptly enrolled in adult education classes. Several of the other women had joined adult education class because they were disconcerted by the apparent disdain which their illiteracy evoked from the more educated members "who are women like ourselves."

Role as Workers

The women recounted many embarrassing work-related experiences which had induced them to enroll in adult education classes. A 38 year-old illiterate trader who sold yams told how she had to pay someone to count them for her. This precluded her ability to expand her business because the more yams she had, the more she had to pay the "yam counter." She felt "degraded" and enrolled in order to "be more educated than my colleagues who helped me count my yams." Another woman's trading business had collapsed due to her nescience of the use of the Ready Reckoner in calculating her transactions, while many other women were unable to count their earnings at the end of each day's work. The seamstresses lamented that their illiteracy was having a deleterious effect on their businesses due to their inability to record their customers' names and sizes and to design the newest styles.

A 41 year-old orange-seller was dysphoric that her best friend's new primary school certificate had secured her an "exciting" cleaning job at the university. She was determined to emulate her friend in using education to obtain a better position. Several other women also regretted having missed an opportunity to be a "civil servant" because when the chance presented itself, they had no primary school certificate.

Another woman, a 36 year-old mother of eight and manager of a small restaurant, recounted the incident which had impelled her to become an adult education student. She had gone to open an account at the bank, dressed in gorgeous attire. When she was offered a pen to sign her name on the form, she requested a stamp pad instead to affix her thumb print since she was illiterate. The acute embarrassment which she experienced when bystanders began snickering left her thoroughly abashed.

Apart from their desire to learn to read, write, calculate, and sign their names, nearly all of the women were anxious to gain fluency in English in order to communicate with non-indigenous customers who account for a good proportion of the population in Nsukka. Others, like the mortified hospital maid who was speechless the day she was asked a question in English by a "top government official," wanted to gain facility in using English in the work place and the office.

Role as Wives and Mothers

Most of the women spoke of their desire to be educated in order to "manage the affairs" of their families better, learn improved health and child rearing practices, recipes for well-balanced meals, family planning methods, etc.

Many of the women had children in both the primary and secondary schools and told of their keen awareness that the children had surpassed them educationally. They longed to have enough education to at least check their children's homework and to take on the teaching of their pre-school children themselves. The 21 year-old mother of a toddler spoke the mind of most of the women when she said she wanted to teach her daughter to read and write and thus "help wipe out illiteracy." This statement points to the fact that a woman's children are often the first to benefit from her education.

The husbands played a prominent role in their wives' education. First of all, the women had obtained their husbands' consent before enrolling, as is customary in the Igbo-speaking areas of Nigeria. Secondly, women who had married men who were more educated than themselves enrolled in adult education to help bridge the gap. They were constantly pinched by the fact that they lacked the educational background to interact confidently with their husbands' colleagues on a social level.

Role as Self-Actualizing Persons

Self-actualization was the underlying motive of the women for enrolling in evening classes in mid-life. They saw adult education as an opportunity to fully develop their potentialities which had been lying dormant for years. As one woman aptly put it, "I am so happy about adult education because I had given up the idea of ever being educated." Others said they wished to "get more knowledge," "to know what is happening in the world," "not to be left behind," "to warm my brain," "to overcome my ignorance," "to be promoted," "to go for further training," "to be learned and be proud of myself," "to read and write personal letters," and "to increase my self-confidence."

BENEFITS DERIVED FROM ADULT EDUCATION

All of the women were eager to describe the ways in which adult education had helped them. Below are some of their comments: "I am improving." "I have achieved a lot." "I am now literate." "I am performing better in trading now and am training others." "I can now identify various chemicals used in hair dressing." "I can read and interpret directions on packets at the ante-natal clinic on how to take drugs." "Adult education has helped me keep my surroundings clean and to cook nutritious meals. My children used to be always sick, but now there is a great improvement." "I can now count my earnings every day." "No one can cheat me now." "After six months of classes, I can count my own yams." "I can read road signs when I travel." "I now keep records in my hairdressing business." "I can write the names of customers who buy on credit." "I now have invoices and I write them myself." "I now behave politely in the meetings instead of shouting people down." "I can measure clothes easier than before." "I am taking the minutes in my town meeting." "I now stand boldly as other women to say something at the meetings." "I am always happy when I remember that I will soon become one of the learned women in my society." "I cannot do without adult education."

THE COSTS OF ATTENDING ADULT EDUCATION

The women narrated ways in which they had completely reorganized their daily schedules in order to attend adult education classes. Most of them woke at 5:00 A.M. to complete all of their domestic tasks before going to work. They also had to close their businesses early so that they could be home to cook supper for their families before the 7:00 P.M. class. Their husbands "refused" to eat food cooked by a child or by any woman other than their wives. This imposed a hardship on many of them, such as the 34 year-old trader who lived a considerable distance from the market, but whose adult education center was near the market premises. After trekking home from her trading activities to prepare the evening meal, it took heroic willpower to trace her steps back again for the evening classes.

The women also reported tensions in their marital relations due to their insistence on attending evening classes. Their husbands "tried to understand" but usually couldn't put up with their wives being gone every evening. Some jealous husbands were enraged if their wives returned a few minutes late. Many, however, were similar to the husband of a 38 year-old trader. She said of him:

> My husband is somebody who has understood the importance of education. He approved right from the first time I mentioned it. He even tries to coach me, although he didn't finish primary school. He hates to see me leaving the house at night. But, due to his appreciation of this program, he has made it a point of duty to come out at the closing hour every day to walk me home.

Childcare was another problem for the women. Some were fortunate in having older children at home to look after the younger ones. Others had no choice but to bundle their infants and toddlers along with them through the dark streets to the class. One woman, whose husband was a night watchman, attended classes infrequently because her husband felt that she should stay at home with their eight children.

The women complained of the high cost of adult education, which, when combined with the exorbitant cost of food, clothes and school fees for their children, imposed on them an additional burden. To save money, most of them had begun the taxing work of home processing the formerly inexpensive family food staples, *gari*, *pap* and *okpa*. The traders added that they often continued working in the market until closing time (6:30) when they had many customers. They hated missing class, but without the extra money from trading, they would have had to drop out of classes.

Despite their willpower and organization, the women said that unforeseen circumstances such as a child's bout with measles, an in-law's death or their own advanced pregnancy, often interrupted their studies. They also struggled with their own "total body weakness" from fulfilling all of their many tasks and sometimes missed classes from sheer exhaustion.

DISCUSSION

This article reported the results of a study of the factors which motivated Nigerian women to attend adult education classes based on their need for role fulfillment.

It was found that most of the women were married, were in their thirties and had between 5 and 8 children. They had missed the opportunity to attend school in their childhood. Nearly half of the women were market traders while others were involved in similar semi-skilled jobs. Most of their husbands were engaged in low level jobs although a few were teachers or university lecturers.

The women were highly motivated to attend adult education classes due to their desire to function optimally in their various roles. They sought to participate fully in social organizations, to be self-reliant in their jobs, to be better managers of their family affairs and to fulfill their need to be knowledgeable and self-directing persons. The classes did meet their self-determined needs and expectations and they made many sacrifices in order to attend them.

For the women in this study, the inability to read, write and count had been a blight on their lives in countless ways. It had barred them from self-respecting interaction with their fellow-women in social organizations. It had made them feel inferior to husbands who were more educated then themselves. It had robbed them of their rightful role as educators of their own children. It had stunted their progress in their occupations, and it had undermined their respect for themselves. It is no surprise, then, that many of them embraced adult education as a powerful means of integrating them with their friends, their families and themselves in healthy and meaningful interaction and in consonance with the full flowering of their many roles.

The 62 women in this study truly appreciated the value of education in helping them fulfill their many roles. It is likely that the 65% of Nigerian women who are estimated to be illiterate (Federal Government of Nigeria, 1987) are also keenly aware of their need for education. Unfortunately, the government's current program for women, known as "Better Life for Rural Women," is totally lacking in educational components. It is instead aimed at enhancing the productive capacity of the masses of rural women in agricultural ventures and remunerative projects, without concurrently raising their educational levels.

The lives of the women in this study were traditional in the extreme. They married young, had many children, were industrious, were expected to cook and cater to their families, and were deferent toward their husbands. The women did not reject these responsibilities. They did, however, use education to transcend them and to gain personal power and self-respect within the cultural matrix in which they found themselves. They sacrificed much in order to attend classes because they realized that adult education was capable of truly liberating them to fulfill their roles and to be all they aspired to be.

REFERENCES

Aubel, J. (1988). Listen then plan: A focus group approach. *Development Communication Report, 60*, 11-14.

Federal Government of Nigeria (1987). *Household surveys of 1987.* Lagos: Federal Ministry of Information Press.

Muganzi, Z. (1988, August). *Focus group discussion method (fgd), a tool for the study of socio-cultural determinants of infant mortality: A case study of Kenya.* Paper presented at the East Africa Workshop on Research and Intervention Issues Concerning Infant and Child Mortality and Health, Dar es Salaam, Tanzania.